THINK**FIT**

7 STEPS TO SETTING INTENTION FOR YOUR HEALTH, WELLNESS, AND MINDSET

ERIC RIAS

Thinkfit: 7 Steps to Setting Intention for Your Health, Wellness, and Mindset

Copyright © 2019 by Eric Rias

Address all inquiries to:
Eric Rias
Email: eric.thinkfitcoach@gmail.com
Website: thinkfitsd.com

Published by:
Kindle Direct Publishing
kdp.amazon.com

Cataloging-in-Publication Data is on file at the Library of Congress

Paperback ISBN: 978-1-09-251292-3

Editor: Tyler Tichelaar, Superior Book Productions
Cover and Interior Design: Fusion Creative Works, fusioncw.com
Writing and Publishing Coach: Christine Gail, christinegail.com
Author Photo: Ashley Sprankles

Every attempt has been made to source properly all quotes.

Printed in the United States of America

TO MY BEAUTIFUL FAMILY:

Micaiah, Isaiah, and my biggest fan, Darla.

You all are my promise.

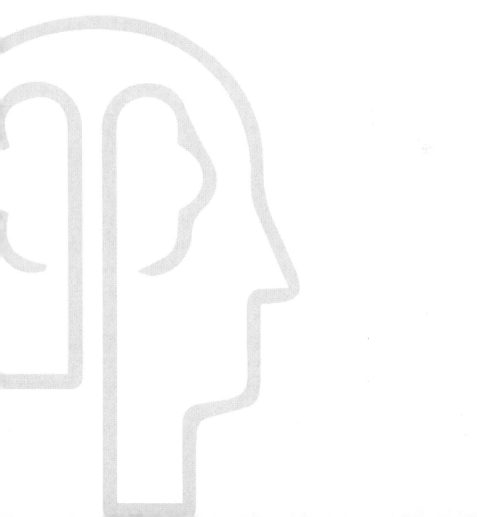

INTRODUCTION

Do we live our lives just "pulling it off"? By pulling it off, I mean that you're hustling, raising children, being a wife or husband, running a business—any or all of the above. This stuff is tough! We wake up every day, pulled by the flow of life's subconscious programming, but maybe that's not working for you anymore. Know that it is possible to wake up every day and really participate in life the way you've always wanted to. To achieve this, I'd like to encourage you to take time to reflect on the twenty-four hours ahead. When you make a conscious effort to *pause*, connect with yourself and others, and set tangible goals, you can achieve more. Through this process, you can set forth ninety days of intentions that can propel you forward beyond the confines of your regularly scheduled programming.

My perspective comes from being a member of a twelve-step program, a personal trainer, and a health coach. The common thread that connects these aspects of my identity is the belief that in order to be successful, I have to seek guidance and take direction when I'm stuck. In my coaching practice when I am working with a client who has hit roadblocks, we create space to reflect and move forward with intention. In this discussion, I will use the term "create space" quite a bit. What that means is allowing and cultivating a cognitive and emotional space of nonjudgment—a place where you can take time to acknowledge your own experience and the intention you'd like to set going forward. This could be eating with intention, planning your day, or accomplishing a purposeful workout, while also creating space to honor yourself. Roadblocks will always be present, but with guidance and the proper steps, it's possible to navigate these obstacles.

I've been stuck many times throughout my life. Growing up and feeling out of place, I developed maladaptive behaviors (to say the least) to cope with life's challenges. Feeling inadequate in an environment where perfectionism thrived led me to many disappointments. My teens and early twenties lacked direction and purpose. Substances helped fill the void of a life that was lacking meaning. Feelings of depression, anxiety, and demoralization governed my life. It was no one else's fault. The life I was creating simply lacked intention. (By intention, I mean I wasn't living a life of purpose that was true to me.) I was in the matrix during this time. Every day felt like Groundhog Day—I would wake up to numb myself, go to some job I didn't want, and spend time with people who didn't care. I had to get desperate in order to change! These feelings I'm describing aren't unique to people afflicted with substance abuse issues. You could be struggling with working a job you aren't fulfilled by or be trapped in an unhealthy relationship that isn't serving you—desperation can come at any time in your life. After a time that I perceived as my pilgrimage through the desert, I found myself desperate enough to ask for help. I became ready to take direction, and I was able to start moving forward.

For five years, I tried many external solutions, hoping they would help me cope with life's ups and downs. I searched for external validation and found no relief. The illusion of validation coming from "things" distorted my view and obscured my purpose. Even sober, I wasn't an active participant in the program of life. Again, I was living in distractions just trying to get to the next day.

Finally, I was presented with a solution that worked for me. I was to start each day with a defined purpose and routine. Waking up with breath, eating a balanced breakfast that nourished my body, and setting personal goals for the day helped propel me forward. I developed a routine of stopping to set an intention for my day and my life. I began a process that enabled me to actively participate in *my* life as opposed to just tolerating regularly scheduled programming. Through these intentions, I've been able to achieve a level of health I never had before. I'm present for my friends and family and have success in reaching my goals.

I believe my life's work is to help others find their way. I don't believe I am special—if I've felt a feeling in the human experience, other people have too. I spent many years of my life believing my feelings were unique to me, but the more I've connected with others and had the opportunity to hear their stories, the more I've realized we are more alike than we are different. So, whether you are a CEO or a newly sober person, we all deserve to live a purposeful life of intention.

A STEP-BY-STEP GUIDE FOR USING THIS BOOK

Now that you are here, you can walk through this process step by step and make it your own. You will have the tools to break through your subconscious programming and set small intentions for each day.

Following are instructions for each step listed on the daily pages to follow so you can easily refer back to these instructions as needed each day.

Before we begin, we must acknowledge the "being intention" and "doing intention." The "being intention" is the state you want to live in. For example, today you want to *live* in compassion, or today you want to *live* in love. The being intention is the state in which we rest for the day. You won't be perfect but setting the day in motion with that intention is a great place to begin. Your "doing intention" is simply a series of action steps to take throughout the day. Cleaning your desk, responding to emails, or completing your workout goal for that day.

Step 1: Upon awakening, you will start by tuning your nervous system for the morning. Our nervous system has two states: parasympathetic and sympathetic. Parasympathetic is our "rest and digest" state, whereas our sympathetic nervous system is our "flight or fight" state. You will use the square breathing technique to manage your nervous system and create the *pause* for your next step.

Step 2: After you've grounded yourself and created breath awareness, you can take time to scan your body. As you scan, identify the feelings you may be carrying in your body. You are encouraged to acknowledge a wide array of emotions as opposed to simply happy, mad, and sad. The challenge is to be specific with feeling and create space to honor that emotion without judgment. The feelings you identify can be motivators for the goals you will be setting in the next steps.

Step 3: Now that you've acknowledged your current emotional state, you want to set up to three "being in-tentions." For example, you can set the intention to live in a space of patience with your children or partner. Or you can set the intention to be compassionate as opposed to judgmental for the day. Be creative; this process is your work. You've now created the state of being you'd like to live in. Moving forward with that intention propels you into the steps that follow.

A STEP-BY-STEP GUIDE FOR USING THIS BOOK

Step 4: Next, set your "doing intention" for the day. First, you'll set up to three short-term goals for the day ahead. These goals may be as simple as cleaning and organizing your desk, returning emails, or catching up on old appointments. No matter how small or simple the daily goals are, write them down. Setting short-term action steps helps create focus and incremental progress that moves you through physical and mental blockages.

This book's intention is to teach you how to create space to project the day that's ahead and reflect on the day that's past. This book outlines a ninety-day project for a reason: Setting six-month and one-year goals are amazing and necessary, but it's challenging to track progress and feel a connection to the pursuit and completion of goals in these time frames. By setting a shorter, ninety-day goal, the end is closer in sight, and when you go through the process of writing the *same* goal daily, you connect with it. You sign a daily contract with yourself to make it happen. Your ninety-day goal could be increasing company revenue by a percentage, losing twenty pounds in twelve weeks, or finishing an existing home project. Whatever it may be, writing it daily for ninety days enables you to feel like you can reach out and touch it.

Step 5: You will complete your "doing intentions" by setting a movement goal and a goal to nurture a personal relationship. It's important to take time out of your day to move. Movement can be done anywhere! You can perform movement drills in the office for twenty minutes on your lunch break or walk your dogs for an hour. Taking time to exercise benefits sleep, releases endorphins, reduces stress, increases cognitive function, and provides many other vital benefits.

You may spend your day interacting with people, but are your interactions meaningful? In this step, you are encouraged to take time to *truly* connect with someone in your life. You could set time for lunch with a friend, dinner with family, or going to the park with your children. These can all be opportunities to connect meaningfully with people in your life.

Step 6: To finish up your morning goals, take time to jot down a few sentences. You can write positive affirmations for yourself or create a morning gratitude list. The point is to *be* mindful for a few moments every morning.

Step 7: At the end of your day, review what happened and take an inventory. This process starts with square breathing: breathing out the business of the day and creating space for healthy reflection of the day. Once your nervous system is tuned, review your successes for the day. Take the time to honor yourself and be proud of your accomplishments. The goal of this book is for you simply to *take the time* to live your life, as opposed to just riding the wave. Next, explore the aspects of your day that could have gone better. What blocked you from your successes? Was it you? Was it another person? Explain the challenges that got in your way and assess what you can do differently to handle them better next time. Do you have to review time management? No matter what reasons, problems, or adjustments arise, keep yourself free from judgment. This process is just a way to collect data that helps you set goals for the following day.

Ultimately, this is your work! This guide is simply composed of suggestions, but you are encouraged to be realistic in the goals and intentions you develop because setting attainable goals aids in success. This project's goal is to look forward to the day ahead, set small goals or intentions to break daily programming, and constructively review your day. The flow of life can be daunting, but allowing space to set clear intentions and reflect encourages prioritization. Breathe, get those projects done, start moving, connect with others, and be conscious of the intentions you'll be making. Honor yourself and honor your body! Everyone deserves to live a life of health, dignity, happiness, and freedom.

DAY**01**

DATE: _____

1. Five minutes of Square Breathing

   Four count inhale
   Four count hold
   Four count exhale
   Four count hold

2. Emotional intelligence

   (You are encouraged to acknowledge a wide array of emotions as opposed to simply happy, mad, and sad. The challenge is to be specific with feeling and create space to honor that emotion without judgment.)

   Identify the feeling in your body
   Release emotions not serving you

3. Set up to three *being* intentions

   Example: Spiritual or cognitive intention

   I will live in compassion.
   I will live in tolerance.
   I will speak with love.

   My *being* intentions for today are:

   _____

   _____

   _____

4. Set up to three *doing* intentions

   Example: Three short-term goals for the day

   Today, I will clean the house.
   I will run daily errands.
   I will meditate for ten minutes.

   My *doing* intentions for today are:

   _____

   _____

   _____

   Acknowledge your ninety-day goal:

   _____

   _____

5. Fitness/Movement goal

   Example: *one-hour workout, bike ride, thirty-minute dog walk, swim...*

   My fitness/movement goal for today is:

   _____

   Personal Relationships

   Example: *One action to nurture a personal relationship*

   Lunch with friend/coworker
   Movie with partner
   Park with children

   My plan for today to nurture a personal relationship:

   _____

6. Short reflection for the day

_____
_____
_____
_____
_____

7. Five minutes of Square Breathing

Four count inhale
Four count hold
Four count exhale
Four count hold

Journal one paragraph reflecting upon your day. This is a constructive review. Keep the reflection nonjudgmental.

Example: *Shortcomings and Successes*

I was resentful, selfish, fearful, dishonest.
I was kind, loving, compassionate.
I achieved all my short-term goals but one.

Include: *Where could I have done better? Constructive improvements...*

_____
_____
_____
_____
_____
_____
_____
_____

DAY02

DATE: _____

1. Five minutes of Square Breathing

   Four count inhale
   Four count hold
   Four count exhale
   Four count hold

2. Emotional intelligence

   Identify the feeling in your body
   Release emotions not serving you

3. Set up to three *being* intentions

   Example: Spiritual or cognitive intention

   I will live in compassion.
   I will live in tolerance.
   I will speak with love.

   My *being* intentions for today are:

   _____
   _____
   _____

4. Set up to three *doing* intentions

   Example: Three short-term goals for the day

   Today, I will clean the house.
   I will run daily errands.
   I will meditate for ten minutes.

   My *doing* intentions for today are:

   _____

   _____

   _____

   Acknowledge your ninety-day goal:

   _____

   _____

5. Fitness/Movement goal

   Example: *one-hour workout, bike ride, thirty-minute dog walk, swim...*

   My fitness/movement goal for today is:

   _____

   Personal Relationships

   Example: *One action to nurture a personal relationship*

   Lunch with friend/coworker
   Movie with partner
   Park with children

   My plan for today to nurture a personal relationship:

   _____

6. Short reflection for the day

_____

_____

_____

_____

_____

7. Five minutes of Square Breathing

   Four count inhale
   Four count hold
   Four count exhale
   Four count hold

   Journal one paragraph reflecting upon your day. This is a constructive review. Keep the reflection nonjudgmental.

   Example: *Shortcomings and Successes*

   I was resentful, selfish, fearful, dishonest.
   I was kind, loving, compassionate.
   I achieved all my short-term goals but one.

   Include: *Where could I have done better? Constructive improvements...*

_____

_____

_____

_____

_____

_____

_____

_____

DAY 03

DATE: _____

1. Five minutes of Square Breathing

   Four count inhale
   Four count hold
   Four count exhale
   Four count hold

2. Emotional intelligence

   Identify the feeling in your body
   Release emotions not serving you

3. Set up to three *being* intentions

   Example: Spiritual or cognitive intention

   I will live in compassion.
   I will live in tolerance.
   I will speak with love.

   My *being* intentions for today are:

   _____
   _____
   _____

4. Set up to three *doing* intentions

   Example: Three short-term goals for the day

   Today, I will clean the house.
   I will run daily errands.
   I will meditate for ten minutes.

   My *doing* intentions for today are:

   _____

   _____

   _____

   Acknowledge your ninety-day goal:

   _____

   _____

5. Fitness/Movement goal

   Example: *one-hour workout, bike ride, thirty-minute dog walk, swim...*

   My fitness/movement goal for today is:

   _____

   Personal Relationships

   Example: *One action to nurture a personal relationship*

   Lunch with friend/coworker
   Movie with partner
   Park with children

   My plan for today to nurture a personal relationship:

   _____

6. Short reflection for the day

_____

_____

_____

_____

_____

7. Five minutes of Square Breathing

Four count inhale
Four count hold
Four count exhale
Four count hold

Journal one paragraph reflecting upon your day. This is a constructive review. Keep the reflection nonjudgmental.

Example: *Shortcomings and Successes*

I was resentful, selfish, fearful, dishonest.
I was kind, loving, compassionate.
I achieved all my short-term goals but one.

Include: *Where could I have done better? Constructive improvements...*

_____

_____

_____

_____

_____

_____

_____

DAY04

DATE: _____

1. Five minutes of Square Breathing

   Four count inhale
   Four count hold
   Four count exhale
   Four count hold

2. Emotional intelligence

   Identify the feeling in your body
   Release emotions not serving you

3. Set up to three *being* intentions

   Example: Spiritual or cognitive intention

   I will live in compassion.
   I will live in tolerance.
   I will speak with love.

   My *being* intentions for today are:

   _____

   _____

   _____

DAY 4

4. Set up to three *doing* intentions

   Example: Three short-term goals for the day

   Today, I will clean the house.
   I will run daily errands.
   I will meditate for ten minutes.

   My *doing* intentions for today are:

   _____

   _____

   _____

   Acknowledge your ninety-day goal:

   _____

   _____

5. Fitness/Movement goal

   Example: *one-hour workout, bike ride, thirty-minute dog walk, swim...*

   My fitness/movement goal for today is:

   _____

   Personal Relationships

   Example: *One action to nurture a personal relationship*

   Lunch with friend/coworker
   Movie with partner
   Park with children

   My plan for today to nurture a personal relationship:

   _____

6. Short reflection for the day

_____
_____
_____
_____
_____

7. Five minutes of Square Breathing
   Four count inhale
   Four count hold
   Four count exhale
   Four count hold

   Journal one paragraph reflecting upon your day. This is a constructive review. Keep the reflection nonjudgmental.

   Example: *Shortcomings and Successes*

   I was resentful, selfish, fearful, dishonest.
   I was kind, loving, compassionate.
   I achieved all my short-term goals but one.

   Include: *Where could I have done better? Constructive improvements...*

_____
_____
_____
_____
_____
_____
_____
_____

DAY 5

DAY 05

DATE: _____

1. Five minutes of Square Breathing

   Four count inhale
   Four count hold
   Four count exhale
   Four count hold

2. Emotional intelligence

   Identify the feeling in your body
   Release emotions not serving you

3. Set up to three *being* intentions

   Example: Spiritual or cognitive intention

   I will live in compassion.
   I will live in tolerance.
   I will speak with love.

   My *being* intentions for today are:

   _____
   _____
   _____

4. Set up to three *doing* intentions

   Example: Three short-term goals for the day

   Today, I will clean the house.
   I will run daily errands.
   I will meditate for ten minutes.

   My *doing* intentions for today are:

   _____

   _____

   _____

   Acknowledge your ninety-day goal:

   _____

   _____

5. Fitness/Movement goal

   Example: *one-hour workout, bike ride, thirty-minute dog walk, swim...*

   My fitness/movement goal for today is:

   _____

   Personal Relationships

   Example: *One action to nurture a personal relationship*

   Lunch with friend/coworker
   Movie with partner
   Park with children

   My plan for today to nurture a personal relationship:

   _____

6. Short reflection for the day

---

7. Five minutes of Square Breathing

   Four count inhale
   Four count hold
   Four count exhale
   Four count hold

   Journal one paragraph reflecting upon your day. This is a constructive review. Keep the reflection nonjudgmental.

   Example: *Shortcomings and Successes*

   I was resentful, selfish, fearful, dishonest.
   I was kind, loving, compassionate.
   I achieved all my short-term goals but one.

   Include: *Where could I have done better? Constructive improvements...*

DAY 06

DATE: _____

1. Five minutes of Square Breathing

   Four count inhale
   Four count hold
   Four count exhale
   Four count hold

2. Emotional intelligence

   Identify the feeling in your body
   Release emotions not serving you

3. Set up to three *being* intentions

   Example: Spiritual or cognitive intention

   I will live in compassion.
   I will live in tolerance.
   I will speak with love.

   My *being* intentions for today are:

   _____
   _____
   _____

4. Set up to three *doing* intentions

   Example: Three short-term goals for the day

   Today, I will clean the house.
   I will run daily errands.
   I will meditate for ten minutes.

   My *doing* intentions for today are:

   _____

   _____

   _____

   Acknowledge your ninety-day goal:

   _____

   _____

5. Fitness/Movement goal

   Example: *one-hour workout, bike ride, thirty-minute dog walk, swim...*

   My fitness/movement goal for today is:

   _____

   Personal Relationships

   Example: *One action to nurture a personal relationship*

   Lunch with friend/coworker
   Movie with partner
   Park with children

   My plan for today to nurture a personal relationship:

   _____

6. Short reflection for the day

_____

_____

_____

_____

_____

7. Five minutes of Square Breathing

Four count inhale
Four count hold
Four count exhale
Four count hold

Journal one paragraph reflecting upon your day.
This is a constructive review. Keep the reflection
nonjudgmental.

Example: *Shortcomings and Successes*

I was resentful, selfish, fearful, dishonest.
I was kind, loving, compassionate.
I achieved all my short-term goals but one.

Include: *Where could I have done better? Constructive*
improvements...

_____

_____

_____

_____

_____

_____

_____

_____

DAY 07

DATE: _____

1. Five minutes of Square Breathing

   Four count inhale
   Four count hold
   Four count exhale
   Four count hold

2. Emotional intelligence

   Identify the feeling in your body
   Release emotions not serving you

3. Set up to three *being* intentions

   Example: Spiritual or cognitive intention

   I will live in compassion.
   I will live in tolerance.
   I will speak with love.

   My *being* intentions for today are:

   _____

   _____

   _____

4. Set up to three *doing* intentions

   Example: Three short-term goals for the day

   Today, I will clean the house.
   I will run daily errands.
   I will meditate for ten minutes.

   My *doing* intentions for today are:

   _____

   _____

   _____

   Acknowledge your ninety-day goal:

   _____

   _____

5. Fitness/Movement goal

   Example: *one-hour workout, bike ride, thirty-minute dog walk, swim...*

   My fitness/movement goal for today is:

   _____

   Personal Relationships

   Example: *One action to nurture a personal relationship*

   Lunch with friend/coworker
   Movie with partner
   Park with children

   My plan for today to nurture a personal relationship:

   _____

6. Short reflection for the day

_____
_____
_____
_____
_____

7. Five minutes of Square Breathing

Four count inhale
Four count hold
Four count exhale
Four count hold

Journal one paragraph reflecting upon your day. This is a constructive review. Keep the reflection nonjudgmental.

Example: *Shortcomings and Successes*

I was resentful, selfish, fearful, dishonest.
I was kind, loving, compassionate.
I achieved all my short-term goals but one.

Include: *Where could I have done better? Constructive improvements...*

_____
_____
_____
_____
_____
_____
_____

DAY08

DATE: _____

1. Five minutes of Square Breathing

   Four count inhale
   Four count hold
   Four count exhale
   Four count hold

2. Emotional intelligence

   Identify the feeling in your body
   Release emotions not serving you

3. Set up to three *being* intentions

   Example: Spiritual or cognitive intention

   I will live in compassion.
   I will live in tolerance.
   I will speak with love.

   My *being* intentions for today are:

   _____

   _____

   _____

4. Set up to three *doing* intentions

   Example: Three short-term goals for the day

   Today, I will clean the house.
   I will run daily errands.
   I will meditate for ten minutes.

   My *doing* intentions for today are:

   _____

   _____

   _____

   Acknowledge your ninety-day goal:

   _____

   _____

5. Fitness/Movement goal

   Example: *one-hour workout, bike ride, thirty-minute dog walk, swim...*

   My fitness/movement goal for today is:

   _____

   Personal Relationships

   Example: *One action to nurture a personal relationship*

   Lunch with friend/coworker
   Movie with partner
   Park with children

   My plan for today to nurture a personal relationship:

   _____

6. Short reflection for the day

_____

_____

_____

_____

_____

7. Five minutes of Square Breathing

Four count inhale
Four count hold
Four count exhale
Four count hold

Journal one paragraph reflecting upon your day.
This is a constructive review. Keep the reflection
nonjudgmental.

Example: *Shortcomings and Successes*

I was resentful, selfish, fearful, dishonest.
I was kind, loving, compassionate.
I achieved all my short-term goals but one.

Include: *Where could I have done better? Constructive
improvements...*

_____

_____

_____

_____

_____

_____

_____

DAY 09

DATE: _____

1. Five minutes of Square Breathing

   Four count inhale
   Four count hold
   Four count exhale
   Four count hold

2. Emotional intelligence

   Identify the feeling in your body
   Release emotions not serving you

3. Set up to three *being* intentions

   Example: Spiritual or cognitive intention

   I will live in compassion.
   I will live in tolerance.
   I will speak with love.

   My *being* intentions for today are:

   _____
   _____
   _____

4. Set up to three *doing* intentions

    Example: Three short-term goals for the day

    Today, I will clean the house.
    I will run daily errands.
    I will meditate for ten minutes.

    My *doing* intentions for today are:

    _____

    _____

    _____

    Acknowledge your ninety-day goal:

    _____

    _____

5. Fitness/Movement goal

    Example: *one-hour workout, bike ride, thirty-minute dog walk, swim...*

    My fitness/movement goal for today is:

    _____

    Personal Relationships

    Example: *One action to nurture a personal relationship*

    Lunch with friend/coworker
    Movie with partner
    Park with children

    My plan for today to nurture a personal relationship:

    _____

6. Short reflection for the day

_____
_____
_____
_____
_____

7. Five minutes of Square Breathing

Four count inhale
Four count hold
Four count exhale
Four count hold

Journal one paragraph reflecting upon your day.
This is a constructive review. Keep the reflection
nonjudgmental.

Example: *Shortcomings and Successes*

I was resentful, selfish, fearful, dishonest.
I was kind, loving, compassionate.
I achieved all my short-term goals but one.

Include: *Where could I have done better? Constructive
improvements...*

_____
_____
_____
_____
_____
_____
_____
_____

DAY10

DATE: _____

1. Five minutes of Square Breathing

   Four count inhale
   Four count hold
   Four count exhale
   Four count hold

2. Emotional intelligence

   Identify the feeling in your body
   Release emotions not serving you

3. Set up to three *being* intentions

   Example: Spiritual or cognitive intention

   I will live in compassion.
   I will live in tolerance.
   I will speak with love.

   My *being* intentions for today are:

   _____

   _____

   _____

4. Set up to three *doing* intentions

   Example: Three short-term goals for the day

   Today, I will clean the house.
   I will run daily errands.
   I will meditate for ten minutes.

   My *doing* intentions for today are:

   _____

   _____

   _____

   Acknowledge your ninety-day goal:

   _____

   _____

5. Fitness/Movement goal

   Example: *one-hour workout, bike ride, thirty-minute dog walk, swim...*

   My fitness/movement goal for today is:

   _____

   Personal Relationships

   Example: *One action to nurture a personal relationship*

   Lunch with friend/coworker
   Movie with partner
   Park with children

   My plan for today to nurture a personal relationship:

   _____

6. Short reflection for the day

_____
_____
_____
_____
_____

7. Five minutes of Square Breathing

Four count inhale
Four count hold
Four count exhale
Four count hold

Journal one paragraph reflecting upon your day. This is a constructive review. Keep the reflection nonjudgmental.

Example: *Shortcomings and Successes*

I was resentful, selfish, fearful, dishonest.
I was kind, loving, compassionate.
I achieved all my short-term goals but one.

Include: *Where could I have done better? Constructive improvements...*

_____
_____
_____
_____
_____
_____
_____

DAY11

DATE: _____

1. Five minutes of Square Breathing

   Four count inhale
   Four count hold
   Four count exhale
   Four count hold

2. Emotional intelligence

   Identify the feeling in your body
   Release emotions not serving you

3. Set up to three *being* intentions

   Example: Spiritual or cognitive intention

   I will live in compassion.
   I will live in tolerance.
   I will speak with love.

   My *being* intentions for today are:

   _____

   _____

   _____

4. Set up to three *doing* intentions

   Example: Three short-term goals for the day

   Today, I will clean the house.
   I will run daily errands.
   I will meditate for ten minutes.

   My *doing* intentions for today are:

   _____

   _____

   _____

   Acknowledge your ninety-day goal:

   _____

   _____

5. Fitness/Movement goal

   Example: *one-hour workout, bike ride, thirty-minute dog walk, swim...*

   My fitness/movement goal for today is:

   _____

   Personal Relationships

   Example: *One action to nurture a personal relationship*

   Lunch with friend/coworker
   Movie with partner
   Park with children

   My plan for today to nurture a personal relationship:

   _____

6. Short reflection for the day

_____

_____

_____

_____

_____

7. Five minutes of Square Breathing

Four count inhale
Four count hold
Four count exhale
Four count hold

Journal one paragraph reflecting upon your day. This is a constructive review. Keep the reflection nonjudgmental.

Example: *Shortcomings and Successes*

I was resentful, selfish, fearful, dishonest.
I was kind, loving, compassionate.
I achieved all my short-term goals but one.

Include: *Where could I have done better? Constructive improvements...*

_____

_____

_____

_____

_____

_____

_____

DAY12

DATE: _____

1. Five minutes of Square Breathing

   Four count inhale
   Four count hold
   Four count exhale
   Four count hold

2. Emotional intelligence

   Identify the feeling in your body
   Release emotions not serving you

3. Set up to three *being* intentions

   Example: Spiritual or cognitive intention

   I will live in compassion.
   I will live in tolerance.
   I will speak with love.

   My *being* intentions for today are:

   _____

   _____

   _____

4. Set up to three *doing* intentions

   Example: Three short-term goals for the day

   Today, I will clean the house.
   I will run daily errands.
   I will meditate for ten minutes.

   My *doing* intentions for today are:

   _____

   _____

   _____

   Acknowledge your ninety-day goal:

   _____

   _____

5. Fitness/Movement goal

   Example: *one-hour workout, bike ride, thirty-minute dog walk, swim...*

   My fitness/movement goal for today is:

   _____

   Personal Relationships

   Example: *One action to nurture a personal relationship*

   Lunch with friend/coworker
   Movie with partner
   Park with children

   My plan for today to nurture a personal relationship:

   _____

6. Short reflection for the day

_____

_____

_____

_____

_____

7. Five minutes of Square Breathing

   Four count inhale
   Four count hold
   Four count exhale
   Four count hold

   Journal one paragraph reflecting upon your day. This is a constructive review. Keep the reflection nonjudgmental.

   Example: _Shortcomings and Successes_

   I was resentful, selfish, fearful, dishonest.
   I was kind, loving, compassionate.
   I achieved all my short-term goals but one.

   Include: _Where could I have done better? Constructive improvements..._

   _____

   _____

   _____

   _____

   _____

   _____

   _____

   _____

DAY13

DATE: _____

1. Five minutes of Square Breathing

   Four count inhale
   Four count hold
   Four count exhale
   Four count hold

2. Emotional intelligence

   Identify the feeling in your body
   Release emotions not serving you

3. Set up to three *being* intentions

   Example: Spiritual or cognitive intention

   I will live in compassion.
   I will live in tolerance.
   I will speak with love.

   My *being* intentions for today are:

   _____

   _____

   _____

4. Set up to three *doing* intentions

   Example: Three short-term goals for the day

   Today, I will clean the house.
   I will run daily errands.
   I will meditate for ten minutes.

   My *doing* intentions for today are:

   _____

   _____

   _____

   Acknowledge your ninety-day goal:

   _____

   _____

5. Fitness/Movement goal

   Example: *one-hour workout, bike ride, thirty-minute dog walk, swim...*

   My fitness/movement goal for today is:

   _____

   Personal Relationships

   Example: *One action to nurture a personal relationship*

   Lunch with friend/coworker
   Movie with partner
   Park with children

   My plan for today to nurture a personal relationship:

   _____

6. Short reflection for the day

7. Five minutes of Square Breathing

   Four count inhale
   Four count hold
   Four count exhale
   Four count hold

   Journal one paragraph reflecting upon your day. This is a constructive review. Keep the reflection nonjudgmental.

   Example: *Shortcomings and Successes*

   I was resentful, selfish, fearful, dishonest.
   I was kind, loving, compassionate.
   I achieved all my short-term goals but one.

   Include: *Where could I have done better? Constructive improvements...*

DAY14

DATE: _____

1. Five minutes of Square Breathing

   Four count inhale
   Four count hold
   Four count exhale
   Four count hold

2. Emotional intelligence

   Identify the feeling in your body
   Release emotions not serving you

3. Set up to three *being* intentions

   Example: Spiritual or cognitive intention

   I will live in compassion.
   I will live in tolerance.
   I will speak with love.

   My *being* intentions for today are:

   _____
   _____
   _____

4. Set up to three *doing* intentions

   Example: Three short-term goals for the day

   Today, I will clean the house.
   I will run daily errands.
   I will meditate for ten minutes.

   My *doing* intentions for today are:

   _____

   _____

   _____

   Acknowledge your ninety-day goal:

   _____

   _____

5. Fitness/Movement goal

   Example: *one-hour workout, bike ride, thirty-minute dog walk, swim...*

   My fitness/movement goal for today is:

   _____

   Personal Relationships

   Example: *One action to nurture a personal relationship*

   Lunch with friend/coworker
   Movie with partner
   Park with children

   My plan for today to nurture a personal relationship:

   _____

6. Short reflection for the day

   _____

   _____

   _____

   _____

   _____

7. Five minutes of Square Breathing

   Four count inhale
   Four count hold
   Four count exhale
   Four count hold

   Journal one paragraph reflecting upon your day.
   This is a constructive review. Keep the reflection
   nonjudgmental.

   Example: _Shortcomings and Successes_

   I was resentful, selfish, fearful, dishonest.
   I was kind, loving, compassionate.
   I achieved all my short-term goals but one.

   Include: _Where could I have done better? Constructive_
   improvements...

   _____

   _____

   _____

   _____

   _____

   _____

   _____

   _____

DAY15

DATE: _____

1. Five minutes of Square Breathing

   Four count inhale
   Four count hold
   Four count exhale
   Four count hold

2. Emotional intelligence

   Identify the feeling in your body
   Release emotions not serving you

3. Set up to three *being* intentions

   Example: Spiritual or cognitive intention

   I will live in compassion.
   I will live in tolerance.
   I will speak with love.

   My *being* intentions for today are:

   _____

   _____

   _____

4. Set up to three *doing* intentions

   Example: Three short-term goals for the day

   Today, I will clean the house.
   I will run daily errands.
   I will meditate for ten minutes.

   My *doing* intentions for today are:

   _____

   _____

   _____

   Acknowledge your ninety-day goal:

   _____

   _____

5. Fitness/Movement goal

   Example: *one-hour workout, bike ride, thirty-minute dog walk, swim...*

   My fitness/movement goal for today is:

   _____

   Personal Relationships

   Example: *One action to nurture a personal relationship*

   Lunch with friend/coworker
   Movie with partner
   Park with children

   My plan for today to nurture a personal relationship:

   _____

6. Short reflection for the day

_____

_____

_____

_____

_____

7. Five minutes of Square Breathing

   Four count inhale
   Four count hold
   Four count exhale
   Four count hold

   Journal one paragraph reflecting upon your day. This is a constructive review. Keep the reflection nonjudgmental.

   Example: *Shortcomings and Successes*

   I was resentful, selfish, fearful, dishonest.
   I was kind, loving, compassionate.
   I achieved all my short-term goals but one.

   Include: *Where could I have done better? Constructive improvements...*

_____

_____

_____

_____

_____

_____

_____

DAY16

DATE: _____

1. Five minutes of Square Breathing

   Four count inhale
   Four count hold
   Four count exhale
   Four count hold

2. Emotional intelligence

   Identify the feeling in your body
   Release emotions not serving you

3. Set up to three *being* intentions

   Example: Spiritual or cognitive intention

   I will live in compassion.
   I will live in tolerance.
   I will speak with love.

   My *being* intentions for today are:

   _____

   _____

   _____

60

4. Set up to three *doing* intentions

   Example: Three short-term goals for the day

   Today, I will clean the house.
   I will run daily errands.
   I will meditate for ten minutes.

   My *doing* intentions for today are:

   _____

   _____

   _____

   Acknowledge your ninety-day goal:

   _____

   _____

5. Fitness/Movement goal

   Example: *one-hour workout, bike ride, thirty-minute dog walk, swim...*

   My fitness/movement goal for today is:

   _____

   Personal Relationships

   Example: *One action to nurture a personal relationship*

   Lunch with friend/coworker
   Movie with partner
   Park with children

   My plan for today to nurture a personal relationship:

   _____

6. Short reflection for the day

_____

_____

_____

_____

_____

7. Five minutes of Square Breathing

Four count inhale
Four count hold
Four count exhale
Four count hold

Journal one paragraph reflecting upon your day.
This is a constructive review. Keep the reflection
nonjudgmental.

Example: *Shortcomings and Successes*

I was resentful, selfish, fearful, dishonest.
I was kind, loving, compassionate.
I achieved all my short-term goals but one.

Include: *Where could I have done better? Constructive
improvements...*

_____

_____

_____

_____

_____

_____

_____

_____

DAY17

DATE: _____

1. Five minutes of Square Breathing

   Four count inhale
   Four count hold
   Four count exhale
   Four count hold

2. Emotional intelligence

   Identify the feeling in your body
   Release emotions not serving you

3. Set up to three *being* intentions

   Example: Spiritual or cognitive intention

   I will live in compassion.
   I will live in tolerance.
   I will speak with love.

   My *being* intentions for today are:

   _____

   _____

   _____

4. Set up to three *doing* intentions

    Example: Three short-term goals for the day

    Today, I will clean the house.
    I will run daily errands.
    I will meditate for ten minutes.

    My *doing* intentions for today are:

    _____

    _____

    _____

    Acknowledge your ninety-day goal:

    _____

    _____

5. Fitness/Movement goal

    Example: *one-hour workout, bike ride, thirty-minute dog walk, swim...*

    My fitness/movement goal for today is:

    _____

    Personal Relationships

    Example: *One action to nurture a personal relationship*

    Lunch with friend/coworker
    Movie with partner
    Park with children

    My plan for today to nurture a personal relationship:

    _____

6. Short reflection for the day

_____

_____

_____

_____

_____

7. Five minutes of Square Breathing

Four count inhale
Four count hold
Four count exhale
Four count hold

Journal one paragraph reflecting upon your day. This is a constructive review. Keep the reflection nonjudgmental.

Example: *Shortcomings and Successes*

I was resentful, selfish, fearful, dishonest.
I was kind, loving, compassionate.
I achieved all my short-term goals but one.

Include: *Where could I have done better? Constructive improvements...*

_____

_____

_____

_____

_____

_____

_____

_____

DAY18

DATE: _____

1. Five minutes of Square Breathing

   Four count inhale
   Four count hold
   Four count exhale
   Four count hold

2. Emotional intelligence

   Identify the feeling in your body
   Release emotions not serving you

3. Set up to three *being* intentions

   Example: Spiritual or cognitive intention

   I will live in compassion.
   I will live in tolerance.
   I will speak with love.

   My *being* intentions for today are:

   _____
   _____
   _____

4. Set up to three *doing* intentions

   Example: Three short-term goals for the day

   Today, I will clean the house.
   I will run daily errands.
   I will meditate for ten minutes.

   My *doing* intentions for today are:

   _____
   _____
   _____

   Acknowledge your ninety-day goal:

   _____
   _____

5. Fitness/Movement goal

   Example: *one-hour workout, bike ride, thirty-minute dog walk, swim...*

   My fitness/movement goal for today is:

   _____

   Personal Relationships

   Example: *One action to nurture a personal relationship*

   Lunch with friend/coworker
   Movie with partner
   Park with children

   My plan for today to nurture a personal relationship:

   _____

6. Short reflection for the day

_____
_____
_____
_____
_____

7. Five minutes of Square Breathing

   Four count inhale
   Four count hold
   Four count exhale
   Four count hold

   Journal one paragraph reflecting upon your day. This is a constructive review. Keep the reflection nonjudgmental.

   Example: _Shortcomings and Successes_

   I was resentful, selfish, fearful, dishonest.
   I was kind, loving, compassionate.
   I achieved all my short-term goals but one.

   Include: _Where could I have done better? Constructive improvements..._

_____
_____
_____
_____
_____
_____
_____

DAY19

DATE: _____

1. Five minutes of Square Breathing

   Four count inhale
   Four count hold
   Four count exhale
   Four count hold

2. Emotional intelligence

   Identify the feeling in your body
   Release emotions not serving you

3. Set up to three *being* intentions

   Example: Spiritual or cognitive intention

   I will live in compassion.
   I will live in tolerance.
   I will speak with love.

   My *being* intentions for today are:

   _____

   _____

   _____

4. Set up to three *doing* intentions

   Example: Three short-term goals for the day

   Today, I will clean the house.
   I will run daily errands.
   I will meditate for ten minutes.

   My *doing* intentions for today are:

   _____

   _____

   _____

   Acknowledge your ninety-day goal:

   _____

   _____

5. Fitness/Movement goal

   Example: *one-hour workout, bike ride, thirty-minute dog walk, swim...*

   My fitness/movement goal for today is:

   _____

   Personal Relationships

   Example: *One action to nurture a personal relationship*

   Lunch with friend/coworker
   Movie with partner
   Park with children

   My plan for today to nurture a personal relationship:

   _____

6. Short reflection for the day

---

7. Five minutes of Square Breathing

   Four count inhale
   Four count hold
   Four count exhale
   Four count hold

   Journal one paragraph reflecting upon your day. This is a constructive review. Keep the reflection nonjudgmental.

   Example: *Shortcomings and Successes*

   I was resentful, selfish, fearful, dishonest.
   I was kind, loving, compassionate.
   I achieved all my short-term goals but one.

   Include: *Where could I have done better? Constructive improvements...*

DAY 20

DATE: _____

1. Five minutes of Square Breathing

   Four count inhale
   Four count hold
   Four count exhale
   Four count hold

2. Emotional intelligence

   Identify the feeling in your body
   Release emotions not serving you

3. Set up to three *being* intentions

   Example: Spiritual or cognitive intention

   I will live in compassion.
   I will live in tolerance.
   I will speak with love.

   My *being* intentions for today are:

   _____
   _____
   _____

4. Set up to three *doing* intentions

   Example: Three short-term goals for the day

   Today, I will clean the house.
   I will run daily errands.
   I will meditate for ten minutes.

   My *doing* intentions for today are:

   _____
   _____
   _____

   Acknowledge your ninety-day goal:

   _____
   _____

5. Fitness/Movement goal

   Example: *one-hour workout, bike ride, thirty-minute dog walk, swim...*

   My fitness/movement goal for today is:

   _____

   Personal Relationships

   Example: *One action to nurture a personal relationship*

   Lunch with friend/coworker
   Movie with partner
   Park with children

   My plan for today to nurture a personal relationship:

   _____

6. Short reflection for the day

_____

_____

_____

_____

_____

7. Five minutes of Square Breathing

Four count inhale
Four count hold
Four count exhale
Four count hold

Journal one paragraph reflecting upon your day. This is a constructive review. Keep the reflection nonjudgmental.

Example: *Shortcomings and Successes*

I was resentful, selfish, fearful, dishonest.
I was kind, loving, compassionate.
I achieved all my short-term goals but one.

Include: *Where could I have done better? Constructive improvements...*

_____

_____

_____

_____

_____

_____

_____

DAY 21

DATE: _____

1. Five minutes of Square Breathing

   Four count inhale
   Four count hold
   Four count exhale
   Four count hold

2. Emotional intelligence

   Identify the feeling in your body
   Release emotions not serving you

3. Set up to three *being* intentions

   Example: Spiritual or cognitive intention

   I will live in compassion.
   I will live in tolerance.
   I will speak with love.

   My *being* intentions for today are:

   _____
   _____
   _____

4. Set up to three *doing* intentions

   Example: Three short-term goals for the day

   Today, I will clean the house.
   I will run daily errands.
   I will meditate for ten minutes.

   My *doing* intentions for today are:

   _____
   _____
   _____

   Acknowledge your ninety-day goal:

   _____
   _____

5. Fitness/Movement goal

   Example: *one-hour workout, bike ride, thirty-minute dog walk, swim...*

   My fitness/movement goal for today is:

   _____

   Personal Relationships

   Example: *One action to nurture a personal relationship*

   Lunch with friend/coworker
   Movie with partner
   Park with children

   My plan for today to nurture a personal relationship:

   _____

6. Short reflection for the day

_____

_____

_____

_____

_____

7. Five minutes of Square Breathing

   Four count inhale
   Four count hold
   Four count exhale
   Four count hold

   Journal one paragraph reflecting upon your day.
   This is a constructive review. Keep the reflection
   nonjudgmental.

   Example: *Shortcomings and Successes*

   I was resentful, selfish, fearful, dishonest.
   I was kind, loving, compassionate.
   I achieved all my short-term goals but one.

   Include: *Where could I have done better? Constructive*
   improvements...

   _____

   _____

   _____

   _____

   _____

   _____

   _____

DAY 22

DATE: _____

1. Five minutes of Square Breathing

   Four count inhale
   Four count hold
   Four count exhale
   Four count hold

2. Emotional intelligence

   Identify the feeling in your body
   Release emotions not serving you

3. Set up to three *being* intentions

   Example: Spiritual or cognitive intention

   I will live in compassion.
   I will live in tolerance.
   I will speak with love.

   My *being* intentions for today are:

   _____
   _____
   _____

4. Set up to three *doing* intentions

    Example: Three short-term goals for the day

    Today, I will clean the house.
    I will run daily errands.
    I will meditate for ten minutes.

    My *doing* intentions for today are:

    _____
    _____
    _____

    Acknowledge your ninety-day goal:

    _____
    _____

5. Fitness/Movement goal

    Example: *one-hour workout, bike ride, thirty-minute dog walk, swim...*

    My fitness/movement goal for today is:

    _____

    Personal Relationships

    Example: *One action to nurture a personal relationship*

    Lunch with friend/coworker
    Movie with partner
    Park with children

    My plan for today to nurture a personal relationship:

    _____

6. Short reflection for the day

_____

_____

_____

_____

_____

7. Five minutes of Square Breathing

Four count inhale
Four count hold
Four count exhale
Four count hold

Journal one paragraph reflecting upon your day. This is a constructive review. Keep the reflection nonjudgmental.

Example: _Shortcomings and Successes_

I was resentful, selfish, fearful, dishonest.
I was kind, loving, compassionate.
I achieved all my short-term goals but one.

Include: _Where could I have done better? Constructive improvements..._

_____

_____

_____

_____

_____

_____

_____

_____

DAY23

DATE: _____

1. Five minutes of Square Breathing

   Four count inhale
   Four count hold
   Four count exhale
   Four count hold

2. Emotional intelligence

   Identify the feeling in your body
   Release emotions not serving you

3. Set up to three *being* intentions

   Example: Spiritual or cognitive intention

   I will live in compassion.
   I will live in tolerance.
   I will speak with love.

   My *being* intentions for today are:

   _____
   _____
   _____

4. Set up to three *doing* intentions

   Example: Three short-term goals for the day

   Today, I will clean the house.
   I will run daily errands.
   I will meditate for ten minutes.

   My *doing* intentions for today are:

   _____

   _____

   _____

   Acknowledge your ninety-day goal:

   _____

   _____

5. Fitness/Movement goal

   Example: *one-hour workout, bike ride, thirty-minute dog walk, swim...*

   My fitness/movement goal for today is:

   _____

   Personal Relationships

   Example: *One action to nurture a personal relationship*

   Lunch with friend/coworker
   Movie with partner
   Park with children

   My plan for today to nurture a personal relationship:

   _____

6. Short reflection for the day

_____

_____

_____

_____

_____

7. Five minutes of Square Breathing

Four count inhale
Four count hold
Four count exhale
Four count hold

Journal one paragraph reflecting upon your day. This is a constructive review. Keep the reflection nonjudgmental.

Example: *Shortcomings and Successes*

I was resentful, selfish, fearful, dishonest.
I was kind, loving, compassionate.
I achieved all my short-term goals but one.

Include: *Where could I have done better? Constructive improvements...*

_____

_____

_____

_____

_____

_____

_____

DAY 24

DATE: _____

1. Five minutes of Square Breathing

   Four count inhale
   Four count hold
   Four count exhale
   Four count hold

2. Emotional intelligence

   Identify the feeling in your body
   Release emotions not serving you

3. Set up to three *being* intentions

   Example: Spiritual or cognitive intention

   I will live in compassion.
   I will live in tolerance.
   I will speak with love.

   My *being* intentions for today are:

   _____
   _____
   _____

4. Set up to three *doing* intentions

   Example: Three short-term goals for the day

   Today, I will clean the house.
   I will run daily errands.
   I will meditate for ten minutes.

   My *doing* intentions for today are:

   _____

   _____

   _____

   Acknowledge your ninety-day goal:

   _____

   _____

5. Fitness/Movement goal

   Example: *one-hour workout, bike ride, thirty-minute dog walk, swim...*

   My fitness/movement goal for today is:

   _____

   Personal Relationships

   Example: *One action to nurture a personal relationship*

   Lunch with friend/coworker
   Movie with partner
   Park with children

   My plan for today to nurture a personal relationship:

   _____

6. Short reflection for the day

_____

_____

_____

_____

_____

7. Five minutes of Square Breathing

Four count inhale
Four count hold
Four count exhale
Four count hold

Journal one paragraph reflecting upon your day. This is a constructive review. Keep the reflection nonjudgmental.

Example: *Shortcomings and Successes*

I was resentful, selfish, fearful, dishonest.
I was kind, loving, compassionate.
I achieved all my short-term goals but one.

Include: *Where could I have done better? Constructive improvements...*

_____

_____

_____

_____

_____

_____

_____

_____

DAY 25

DATE: _____

1. Five minutes of Square Breathing

   Four count inhale
   Four count hold
   Four count exhale
   Four count hold

2. Emotional intelligence

   Identify the feeling in your body
   Release emotions not serving you

3. Set up to three *being* intentions

   Example: Spiritual or cognitive intention

   I will live in compassion.
   I will live in tolerance.
   I will speak with love.

   My *being* intentions for today are:

   _____

   _____

   _____

4. Set up to three *doing* intentions

    Example: Three short-term goals for the day

    Today, I will clean the house.
    I will run daily errands.
    I will meditate for ten minutes.

    My *doing* intentions for today are:

    _____

    _____

    _____

    Acknowledge your ninety-day goal:

    _____

    _____

5. Fitness/Movement goal

    Example: *one-hour workout, bike ride, thirty-minute dog walk, swim...*

    My fitness/movement goal for today is:

    _____

    Personal Relationships

    Example: *One action to nurture a personal relationship*

    Lunch with friend/coworker
    Movie with partner
    Park with children

    My plan for today to nurture a personal relationship:

    _____

6. Short reflection for the day

_____
_____
_____
_____
_____

7. Five minutes of Square Breathing

Four count inhale
Four count hold
Four count exhale
Four count hold

Journal one paragraph reflecting upon your day. This is a constructive review. Keep the reflection nonjudgmental.

Example: *Shortcomings and Successes*

I was resentful, selfish, fearful, dishonest.
I was kind, loving, compassionate.
I achieved all my short-term goals but one.

Include: *Where could I have done better? Constructive improvements...*

_____
_____
_____
_____
_____
_____
_____
_____

DAY26

DATE: _____

1. Five minutes of Square Breathing

   Four count inhale
   Four count hold
   Four count exhale
   Four count hold

2. Emotional intelligence

   Identify the feeling in your body
   Release emotions not serving you

3. Set up to three *being* intentions

   Example: Spiritual or cognitive intention

   I will live in compassion.
   I will live in tolerance.
   I will speak with love.

   My *being* intentions for today are:

   _____
   _____
   _____

4. Set up to three *doing* intentions

   Example: Three short-term goals for the day

   Today, I will clean the house.
   I will run daily errands.
   I will meditate for ten minutes.

   My *doing* intentions for today are:

   _____

   _____

   _____

   Acknowledge your ninety-day goal:

   _____

   _____

5. Fitness/Movement goal

   Example: *one-hour workout, bike ride, thirty-minute dog walk, swim...*

   My fitness/movement goal for today is:

   _____

   Personal Relationships

   Example: *One action to nurture a personal relationship*

   Lunch with friend/coworker
   Movie with partner
   Park with children

   My plan for today to nurture a personal relationship:

   _____

6. Short reflection for the day

_____

_____

_____

_____

_____

7. Five minutes of Square Breathing

    Four count inhale
    Four count hold
    Four count exhale
    Four count hold

    Journal one paragraph reflecting upon your day.
    This is a constructive review. Keep the reflection
    nonjudgmental.

    Example: _Shortcomings and Successes_

    I was resentful, selfish, fearful, dishonest.
    I was kind, loving, compassionate.
    I achieved all my short-term goals but one.

    Include: _Where could I have done better? Constructive_
    improvements...

_____

_____

_____

_____

_____

_____

_____

_____

DAY27

DATE: _____

1. Five minutes of Square Breathing

   Four count inhale
   Four count hold
   Four count exhale
   Four count hold

2. Emotional intelligence

   Identify the feeling in your body
   Release emotions not serving you

3. Set up to three *being* intentions

   Example: Spiritual or cognitive intention

   I will live in compassion.
   I will live in tolerance.
   I will speak with love.

   My *being* intentions for today are:

   _____
   _____
   _____

4. Set up to three *doing* intentions

   Example: Three short-term goals for the day

   Today, I will clean the house.
   I will run daily errands.
   I will meditate for ten minutes.

   My *doing* intentions for today are:

   _____

   _____

   _____

   Acknowledge your ninety-day goal:

   _____

   _____

5. Fitness/Movement goal

   Example: *one-hour workout, bike ride, thirty-minute dog walk, swim...*

   My fitness/movement goal for today is:

   _____

   Personal Relationships

   Example: *One action to nurture a personal relationship*

   Lunch with friend/coworker
   Movie with partner
   Park with children

   My plan for today to nurture a personal relationship:

   _____

6. Short reflection for the day

_____

_____

_____

_____

_____

7. Five minutes of Square Breathing

Four count inhale
Four count hold
Four count exhale
Four count hold

Journal one paragraph reflecting upon your day.
This is a constructive review. Keep the reflection
nonjudgmental.

Example: *Shortcomings and Successes*

I was resentful, selfish, fearful, dishonest.
I was kind, loving, compassionate.
I achieved all my short-term goals but one.

Include: *Where could I have done better? Constructive
improvements...*

_____

_____

_____

_____

_____

_____

_____

DAY 28

DATE: _____

1. Five minutes of Square Breathing

   Four count inhale
   Four count hold
   Four count exhale
   Four count hold

2. Emotional intelligence

   Identify the feeling in your body
   Release emotions not serving you

3. Set up to three *being* intentions

   Example: Spiritual or cognitive intention

   I will live in compassion.
   I will live in tolerance.
   I will speak with love.

   My *being* intentions for today are:

   _____
   _____
   _____

DAY 28

4. Set up to three *doing* intentions

   Example: Three short-term goals for the day

   Today, I will clean the house.
   I will run daily errands.
   I will meditate for ten minutes.

   My *doing* intentions for today are:

   _____
   _____
   _____

   Acknowledge your ninety-day goal:

   _____
   _____

5. Fitness/Movement goal

   Example: *one-hour workout, bike ride, thirty-minute dog walk, swim...*

   My fitness/movement goal for today is:

   _____

   Personal Relationships

   Example: *One action to nurture a personal relationship*

   Lunch with friend/coworker
   Movie with partner
   Park with children

   My plan for today to nurture a personal relationship:

   _____

6. Short reflection for the day

---

7. Five minutes of Square Breathing

   Four count inhale
   Four count hold
   Four count exhale
   Four count hold

   Journal one paragraph reflecting upon your day. This is a constructive review. Keep the reflection nonjudgmental.

   Example: *Shortcomings and Successes*

   I was resentful, selfish, fearful, dishonest.
   I was kind, loving, compassionate.
   I achieved all my short-term goals but one.

   Include: *Where could I have done better? Constructive improvements...*

DAY29

DATE: _____

1. Five minutes of Square Breathing

   Four count inhale
   Four count hold
   Four count exhale
   Four count hold

2. Emotional intelligence

   Identify the feeling in your body
   Release emotions not serving you

3. Set up to three *being* intentions

   Example: Spiritual or cognitive intention

   I will live in compassion.
   I will live in tolerance.
   I will speak with love.

   My *being* intentions for today are:

   _____
   _____
   _____

4. Set up to three *doing* intentions

   Example: Three short-term goals for the day

   Today, I will clean the house.
   I will run daily errands.
   I will meditate for ten minutes.

   My *doing* intentions for today are:

   _____

   _____

   _____

   Acknowledge your ninety-day goal:

   _____

   _____

5. Fitness/Movement goal

   Example: *one-hour workout, bike ride, thirty-minute dog walk, swim...*

   My fitness/movement goal for today is:

   _____

   Personal Relationships

   Example: *One action to nurture a personal relationship*

   Lunch with friend/coworker
   Movie with partner
   Park with children

   My plan for today to nurture a personal relationship:

   _____

6. Short reflection for the day

_____
_____
_____
_____
_____

7. Five minutes of Square Breathing

Four count inhale
Four count hold
Four count exhale
Four count hold

Journal one paragraph reflecting upon your day. This is a constructive review. Keep the reflection nonjudgmental.

Example: *Shortcomings and Successes*

I was resentful, selfish, fearful, dishonest.
I was kind, loving, compassionate.
I achieved all my short-term goals but one.

Include: *Where could I have done better? Constructive improvements...*

_____
_____
_____
_____
_____
_____
_____
_____

DAY 30

DATE: _____

1. Five minutes of Square Breathing

   Four count inhale
   Four count hold
   Four count exhale
   Four count hold

2. Emotional intelligence

   Identify the feeling in your body
   Release emotions not serving you

3. Set up to three *being* intentions

   Example: Spiritual or cognitive intention

   I will live in compassion.
   I will live in tolerance.
   I will speak with love.

   My *being* intentions for today are:

   _____
   _____
   _____

4. Set up to three *doing* intentions

   Example: Three short-term goals for the day

   Today, I will clean the house.
   I will run daily errands.
   I will meditate for ten minutes.

   My *doing* intentions for today are:

   _____

   _____

   _____

   Acknowledge your ninety-day goal:

   _____

   _____

5. Fitness/Movement goal

   Example: *one-hour workout, bike ride, thirty-minute dog walk, swim...*

   My fitness/movement goal for today is:

   _____

   Personal Relationships

   Example: *One action to nurture a personal relationship*

   Lunch with friend/coworker
   Movie with partner
   Park with children

   My plan for today to nurture a personal relationship:

   _____

6. Short reflection for the day

   _____

   _____

   _____

   _____

   _____

7. Five minutes of Square Breathing

   Four count inhale
   Four count hold
   Four count exhale
   Four count hold

   Journal one paragraph reflecting upon your day.
   This is a constructive review. Keep the reflection
   nonjudgmental.

   Example: *Shortcomings and Successes*

   I was resentful, selfish, fearful, dishonest.
   I was kind, loving, compassionate.
   I achieved all my short-term goals but one.

   Include: *Where could I have done better? Constructive*
   improvements...

   _____

   _____

   _____

   _____

   _____

   _____

   _____

   _____

DAY 31

DATE: _____

1. Five minutes of Square Breathing

   Four count inhale
   Four count hold
   Four count exhale
   Four count hold

2. Emotional intelligence

   Identify the feeling in your body
   Release emotions not serving you

3. Set up to three *being* intentions

   Example: Spiritual or cognitive intention

   I will live in compassion.
   I will live in tolerance.
   I will speak with love.

   My *being* intentions for today are:

   _____

   _____

   _____

4. Set up to three *doing* intentions

   Example: Three short-term goals for the day

   Today, I will clean the house.
   I will run daily errands.
   I will meditate for ten minutes.

   My *doing* intentions for today are:

   _____
   _____
   _____

   Acknowledge your ninety-day goal:

   _____
   _____

5. Fitness/Movement goal

   Example: *one-hour workout, bike ride, thirty-minute dog walk, swim...*

   My fitness/movement goal for today is:

   _____

   Personal Relationships

   Example: *One action to nurture a personal relationship*

   Lunch with friend/coworker
   Movie with partner
   Park with children

   My plan for today to nurture a personal relationship:

   _____

6. Short reflection for the day

7. Five minutes of Square Breathing

    Four count inhale
    Four count hold
    Four count exhale
    Four count hold

    Journal one paragraph reflecting upon your day. This is a constructive review. Keep the reflection nonjudgmental.

    Example: *Shortcomings and Successes*

    I was resentful, selfish, fearful, dishonest.
    I was kind, loving, compassionate.
    I achieved all my short-term goals but one.

    Include: *Where could I have done better? Constructive improvements...*

DAY 32

DATE: _____

1. Five minutes of Square Breathing

   Four count inhale
   Four count hold
   Four count exhale
   Four count hold

2. Emotional intelligence

   Identify the feeling in your body
   Release emotions not serving you

3. Set up to three *being* intentions

   Example: Spiritual or cognitive intention

   I will live in compassion.
   I will live in tolerance.
   I will speak with love.

   My *being* intentions for today are:

   _____
   _____
   _____

4. Set up to three *doing* intentions

   Example: Three short-term goals for the day

   Today, I will clean the house.
   I will run daily errands.
   I will meditate for ten minutes.

   My *doing* intentions for today are:

   _____
   _____
   _____

   Acknowledge your ninety-day goal:

   _____
   _____

5. Fitness/Movement goal

   Example: *one-hour workout, bike ride, thirty-minute dog walk, swim...*

   My fitness/movement goal for today is:

   _____

   Personal Relationships

   Example: *One action to nurture a personal relationship*

   Lunch with friend/coworker
   Movie with partner
   Park with children

   My plan for today to nurture a personal relationship:

   _____

6. Short reflection for the day

    _____

    _____

    _____

    _____

    _____

7. Five minutes of Square Breathing

   Four count inhale
   Four count hold
   Four count exhale
   Four count hold

   Journal one paragraph reflecting upon your day.
   This is a constructive review. Keep the reflection
   nonjudgmental.

   Example: *Shortcomings and Successes*

   I was resentful, selfish, fearful, dishonest.
   I was kind, loving, compassionate.
   I achieved all my short-term goals but one.

   Include: *Where could I have done better? Constructive*
   improvements...

       _____

       _____

       _____

       _____

       _____

       _____

       _____

       _____

DAY33

DATE: _____

1. Five minutes of Square Breathing

   Four count inhale
   Four count hold
   Four count exhale
   Four count hold

2. Emotional intelligence

   Identify the feeling in your body
   Release emotions not serving you

3. Set up to three *being* intentions

   Example: Spiritual or cognitive intention

   I will live in compassion.
   I will live in tolerance.
   I will speak with love.

   My *being* intentions for today are:

   _____
   _____
   _____

4. Set up to three *doing* intentions

    Example: Three short-term goals for the day

    Today, I will clean the house.
    I will run daily errands.
    I will meditate for ten minutes.

    My *doing* intentions for today are:

    _____
    _____
    _____

    Acknowledge your ninety-day goal:

    _____
    _____

5. Fitness/Movement goal

    Example: *one-hour workout, bike ride, thirty-minute dog walk, swim...*

    My fitness/movement goal for today is:

    _____

    Personal Relationships

    Example: *One action to nurture a personal relationship*

    Lunch with friend/coworker
    Movie with partner
    Park with children

    My plan for today to nurture a personal relationship:

    _____

6. Short reflection for the day

_____

_____

_____

_____

_____

7. Five minutes of Square Breathing

    Four count inhale
    Four count hold
    Four count exhale
    Four count hold

    Journal one paragraph reflecting upon your day. This is a constructive review. Keep the reflection nonjudgmental.

    Example: *Shortcomings and Successes*

    I was resentful, selfish, fearful, dishonest.
    I was kind, loving, compassionate.
    I achieved all my short-term goals but one.

    Include: *Where could I have done better? Constructive improvements...*

_____

_____

_____

_____

_____

_____

_____

_____

DAY 34

DATE: _____

1. Five minutes of Square Breathing

   Four count inhale
   Four count hold
   Four count exhale
   Four count hold

2. Emotional intelligence

   Identify the feeling in your body
   Release emotions not serving you

3. Set up to three *being* intentions

   Example: Spiritual or cognitive intention

   I will live in compassion.
   I will live in tolerance.
   I will speak with love.

   My *being* intentions for today are:

   _____

   _____

   _____

4. Set up to three *doing* intentions

    Example: Three short-term goals for the day

    Today, I will clean the house.
    I will run daily errands.
    I will meditate for ten minutes.

    My *doing* intentions for today are:

    _____
    _____
    _____

    Acknowledge your ninety-day goal:

    _____
    _____

5. Fitness/Movement goal

    Example: *one-hour workout, bike ride, thirty-minute dog walk, swim...*

    My fitness/movement goal for today is:

    _____

    Personal Relationships

    Example: *One action to nurture a personal relationship*

    Lunch with friend/coworker
    Movie with partner
    Park with children

    My plan for today to nurture a personal relationship:

    _____

6. Short reflection for the day

_____

_____

_____

_____

_____

7. Five minutes of Square Breathing

   Four count inhale
   Four count hold
   Four count exhale
   Four count hold

   Journal one paragraph reflecting upon your day. This is a constructive review. Keep the reflection nonjudgmental.

   Example: *Shortcomings and Successes*

   I was resentful, selfish, fearful, dishonest.
   I was kind, loving, compassionate.
   I achieved all my short-term goals but one.

   Include: *Where could I have done better? Constructive improvements...*

_____

_____

_____

_____

_____

_____

_____

DAY 35

DATE: _____

1. Five minutes of Square Breathing

   Four count inhale
   Four count hold
   Four count exhale
   Four count hold

2. Emotional intelligence

   Identify the feeling in your body
   Release emotions not serving you

3. Set up to three *being* intentions

   Example: Spiritual or cognitive intention

   I will live in compassion.
   I will live in tolerance.
   I will speak with love.

   My *being* intentions for today are:

   _____
   _____
   _____

4. Set up to three *doing* intentions

   Example: Three short-term goals for the day

   Today, I will clean the house.
   I will run daily errands.
   I will meditate for ten minutes.

   My *doing* intentions for today are:

   _____
   _____
   _____

   Acknowledge your ninety-day goal:

   _____
   _____

5. Fitness/Movement goal

   Example: *one-hour workout, bike ride, thirty-minute dog walk, swim...*

   My fitness/movement goal for today is:

   _____

   Personal Relationships

   Example: *One action to nurture a personal relationship*

   Lunch with friend/coworker
   Movie with partner
   Park with children

   My plan for today to nurture a personal relationship:

   _____

6. Short reflection for the day

_____

_____

_____

_____

_____

7. Five minutes of Square Breathing

Four count inhale
Four count hold
Four count exhale
Four count hold

Journal one paragraph reflecting upon your day. This is a constructive review. Keep the reflection nonjudgmental.

Example: *Shortcomings and Successes*

I was resentful, selfish, fearful, dishonest.
I was kind, loving, compassionate.
I achieved all my short-term goals but one.

Include: *Where could I have done better? Constructive improvements...*

_____

_____

_____

_____

_____

_____

_____

_____

DAY 36

DATE: _____

1. Five minutes of Square Breathing

   Four count inhale
   Four count hold
   Four count exhale
   Four count hold

2. Emotional intelligence

   Identify the feeling in your body
   Release emotions not serving you

3. Set up to three *being* intentions

   Example: Spiritual or cognitive intention

   I will live in compassion.
   I will live in tolerance.
   I will speak with love.

   My *being* intentions for today are:

   _____
   _____
   _____

4. Set up to three *doing* intentions

   Example: Three short-term goals for the day

   Today, I will clean the house.
   I will run daily errands.
   I will meditate for ten minutes.

   My *doing* intentions for today are:

   _____
   _____
   _____

   Acknowledge your ninety-day goal:

   _____
   _____

5. Fitness/Movement goal

   Example: *one-hour workout, bike ride, thirty-minute dog walk, swim...*

   My fitness/movement goal for today is:

   _____

   Personal Relationships

   Example: *One action to nurture a personal relationship*

   Lunch with friend/coworker
   Movie with partner
   Park with children

   My plan for today to nurture a personal relationship:

   _____

6. Short reflection for the day

    _____

    _____

    _____

    _____

    _____

7. Five minutes of Square Breathing

    Four count inhale
    Four count hold
    Four count exhale
    Four count hold

    Journal one paragraph reflecting upon your day.
    This is a constructive review. Keep the reflection
    nonjudgmental.

    Example: *Shortcomings and Successes*

    I was resentful, selfish, fearful, dishonest.
    I was kind, loving, compassionate.
    I achieved all my short-term goals but one.

    Include: *Where could I have done better? Constructive*
    improvements...

    _____

    _____

    _____

    _____

    _____

    _____

    _____

DAY**37**

DATE: _____

1. Five minutes of Square Breathing

   Four count inhale
   Four count hold
   Four count exhale
   Four count hold

2. Emotional intelligence

   Identify the feeling in your body
   Release emotions not serving you

3. Set up to three *being* intentions

   Example: Spiritual or cognitive intention

   I will live in compassion.
   I will live in tolerance.
   I will speak with love.

   My *being* intentions for today are:

   _____

   _____

   _____

4. Set up to three *doing* intentions

   Example: Three short-term goals for the day

   Today, I will clean the house.
   I will run daily errands.
   I will meditate for ten minutes.

   My *doing* intentions for today are:

   _____
   _____
   _____

   Acknowledge your ninety-day goal:

   _____
   _____

5. Fitness/Movement goal

   Example: *one-hour workout, bike ride, thirty-minute dog walk, swim...*

   My fitness/movement goal for today is:

   _____

   Personal Relationships

   Example: *One action to nurture a personal relationship*

   Lunch with friend/coworker
   Movie with partner
   Park with children

   My plan for today to nurture a personal relationship:

   _____

6. Short reflection for the day

_____
_____
_____
_____
_____

7. Five minutes of Square Breathing

Four count inhale
Four count hold
Four count exhale
Four count hold

Journal one paragraph reflecting upon your day. This is a constructive review. Keep the reflection nonjudgmental.

Example: *Shortcomings and Successes*

I was resentful, selfish, fearful, dishonest.
I was kind, loving, compassionate.
I achieved all my short-term goals but one.

Include: *Where could I have done better? Constructive improvements...*

_____
_____
_____
_____
_____
_____
_____
_____

DAY 38

DATE: _____

1. Five minutes of Square Breathing

   Four count inhale
   Four count hold
   Four count exhale
   Four count hold

2. Emotional intelligence

   Identify the feeling in your body
   Release emotions not serving you

3. Set up to three *being* intentions

   Example: Spiritual or cognitive intention

   I will live in compassion.
   I will live in tolerance.
   I will speak with love.

   My *being* intentions for today are:

   _____
   _____
   _____

4. Set up to three *doing* intentions

   Example: Three short-term goals for the day

   Today, I will clean the house.
   I will run daily errands.
   I will meditate for ten minutes.

   My *doing* intentions for today are:

   _____
   _____
   _____

   Acknowledge your ninety-day goal:

   _____
   _____

5. Fitness/Movement goal

   Example: *one-hour workout, bike ride, thirty-minute dog walk, swim...*

   My fitness/movement goal for today is:

   _____

   Personal Relationships

   Example: *One action to nurture a personal relationship*

   Lunch with friend/coworker
   Movie with partner
   Park with children

   My plan for today to nurture a personal relationship:

   _____

6. Short reflection for the day

_____
_____
_____
_____
_____

7. Five minutes of Square Breathing
    Four count inhale
    Four count hold
    Four count exhale
    Four count hold

    Journal one paragraph reflecting upon your day.
    This is a constructive review. Keep the reflection
    nonjudgmental.

    Example: *Shortcomings and Successes*

    I was resentful, selfish, fearful, dishonest.
    I was kind, loving, compassionate.
    I achieved all my short-term goals but one.

    Include: *Where could I have done better? Constructive*
    improvements...

_____
_____
_____
_____
_____
_____
_____
_____

DAY 39

DATE: _____

1. Five minutes of Square Breathing

   Four count inhale
   Four count hold
   Four count exhale
   Four count hold

2. Emotional intelligence

   Identify the feeling in your body
   Release emotions not serving you

3. Set up to three *being* intentions

   Example: Spiritual or cognitive intention

   I will live in compassion.
   I will live in tolerance.
   I will speak with love.

   My *being* intentions for today are:

   _____

   _____

   _____

4. Set up to three *doing* intentions

   Example: Three short-term goals for the day

   Today, I will clean the house.
   I will run daily errands.
   I will meditate for ten minutes.

   My *doing* intentions for today are:

   _____
   _____
   _____

   Acknowledge your ninety-day goal:

   _____
   _____

5. Fitness/Movement goal

   Example: *one-hour workout, bike ride, thirty-minute dog walk, swim...*

   My fitness/movement goal for today is:

   _____

   Personal Relationships

   Example: *One action to nurture a personal relationship*

   Lunch with friend/coworker
   Movie with partner
   Park with children

   My plan for today to nurture a personal relationship:

   _____

6. Short reflection for the day

_____

_____

_____

_____

_____

7. Five minutes of Square Breathing

Four count inhale
Four count hold
Four count exhale
Four count hold

Journal one paragraph reflecting upon your day. This is a constructive review. Keep the reflection nonjudgmental.

Example: *Shortcomings and Successes*

I was resentful, selfish, fearful, dishonest.
I was kind, loving, compassionate.
I achieved all my short-term goals but one.

Include: *Where could I have done better? Constructive improvements…*

_____

_____

_____

_____

_____

_____

_____

_____

DAY 40

DATE: _____

1. Five minutes of Square Breathing

   Four count inhale
   Four count hold
   Four count exhale
   Four count hold

2. Emotional intelligence

   Identify the feeling in your body
   Release emotions not serving you

3. Set up to three *being* intentions

   Example: Spiritual or cognitive intention

   I will live in compassion.
   I will live in tolerance.
   I will speak with love.

   My *being* intentions for today are:

   _____
   _____
   _____

4. Set up to three *doing* intentions

   Example: Three short-term goals for the day

   Today, I will clean the house.
   I will run daily errands.
   I will meditate for ten minutes.

   My *doing* intentions for today are:

   _____

   _____

   _____

   Acknowledge your ninety-day goal:

   _____

   _____

5. Fitness/Movement goal

   Example: *one-hour workout, bike ride, thirty-minute dog walk, swim...*

   My fitness/movement goal for today is:

   _____

   Personal Relationships

   Example: *One action to nurture a personal relationship*

   Lunch with friend/coworker
   Movie with partner
   Park with children

   My plan for today to nurture a personal relationship:

   _____

6. Short reflection for the day

_____

_____

_____

_____

_____

7. Five minutes of Square Breathing

Four count inhale
Four count hold
Four count exhale
Four count hold

Journal one paragraph reflecting upon your day. This is a constructive review. Keep the reflection nonjudgmental.

Example: *Shortcomings and Successes*

I was resentful, selfish, fearful, dishonest.
I was kind, loving, compassionate.
I achieved all my short-term goals but one.

Include: *Where could I have done better? Constructive improvements...*

_____

_____

_____

_____

_____

_____

_____

_____

DAY 41

DATE: _____

1. Five minutes of Square Breathing

   Four count inhale
   Four count hold
   Four count exhale
   Four count hold

2. Emotional intelligence

   Identify the feeling in your body
   Release emotions not serving you

3. Set up to three *being* intentions

   Example: Spiritual or cognitive intention

   I will live in compassion.
   I will live in tolerance.
   I will speak with love.

   My *being* intentions for today are:

   _____
   _____
   _____

135

4. Set up to three *doing* intentions

   Example: Three short-term goals for the day

   Today, I will clean the house.
   I will run daily errands.
   I will meditate for ten minutes.

   My *doing* intentions for today are:

   _____

   _____

   _____

   Acknowledge your ninety-day goal:

   _____

   _____

5. Fitness/Movement goal

   Example: *one-hour workout, bike ride, thirty-minute dog walk, swim...*

   My fitness/movement goal for today is:

   _____

   Personal Relationships

   Example: *One action to nurture a personal relationship*

   Lunch with friend/coworker
   Movie with partner
   Park with children

   My plan for today to nurture a personal relationship:

   _____

6. Short reflection for the day

_____

_____

_____

_____

_____

7. Five minutes of Square Breathing

Four count inhale
Four count hold
Four count exhale
Four count hold

Journal one paragraph reflecting upon your day. This is a constructive review. Keep the reflection nonjudgmental.

Example: *Shortcomings and Successes*

I was resentful, selfish, fearful, dishonest.
I was kind, loving, compassionate.
I achieved all my short-term goals but one.

Include: *Where could I have done better? Constructive improvements...*

_____

_____

_____

_____

_____

_____

_____

DAY 42

DATE: _____

1. Five minutes of Square Breathing

   Four count inhale
   Four count hold
   Four count exhale
   Four count hold

2. Emotional intelligence

   Identify the feeling in your body
   Release emotions not serving you

3. Set up to three *being* intentions

   Example: Spiritual or cognitive intention

   I will live in compassion.
   I will live in tolerance.
   I will speak with love.

   My *being* intentions for today are:

   _____
   _____
   _____

4. Set up to three *doing* intentions

   Example: Three short-term goals for the day

   Today, I will clean the house.
   I will run daily errands.
   I will meditate for ten minutes.

   My *doing* intentions for today are:

   _____

   _____

   _____

   Acknowledge your ninety-day goal:

   _____

   _____

5. Fitness/Movement goal

   Example: *one-hour workout, bike ride, thirty-minute dog walk, swim...*

   My fitness/movement goal for today is:

   _____

   Personal Relationships

   Example: *One action to nurture a personal relationship*

   Lunch with friend/coworker
   Movie with partner
   Park with children

   My plan for today to nurture a personal relationship:

   _____

6. Short reflection for the day

_____

_____

_____

_____

_____

7. Five minutes of Square Breathing

Four count inhale
Four count hold
Four count exhale
Four count hold

Journal one paragraph reflecting upon your day. This is a constructive review. Keep the reflection nonjudgmental.

Example: *Shortcomings and Successes*

I was resentful, selfish, fearful, dishonest.
I was kind, loving, compassionate.
I achieved all my short-term goals but one.

Include: *Where could I have done better? Constructive improvements...*

_____

_____

_____

_____

_____

_____

_____

_____

DAY 43

DATE: _____

1. Five minutes of Square Breathing

   Four count inhale
   Four count hold
   Four count exhale
   Four count hold

2. Emotional intelligence

   Identify the feeling in your body
   Release emotions not serving you

3. Set up to three *being* intentions

   Example: Spiritual or cognitive intention

   I will live in compassion.
   I will live in tolerance.
   I will speak with love.

   My *being* intentions for today are:

   _____
   _____
   _____

4. Set up to three *doing* intentions

   Example: Three short-term goals for the day

   Today, I will clean the house.
   I will run daily errands.
   I will meditate for ten minutes.

   My *doing* intentions for today are:

   _____
   _____
   _____

   Acknowledge your ninety-day goal:

   _____
   _____

5. Fitness/Movement goal

   Example: *one-hour workout, bike ride, thirty-minute dog walk, swim...*

   My fitness/movement goal for today is:

   _____

   Personal Relationships

   Example: *One action to nurture a personal relationship*

   Lunch with friend/coworker
   Movie with partner
   Park with children

   My plan for today to nurture a personal relationship:

   _____

6. Short reflection for the day

_____

_____

_____

_____

_____

7. Five minutes of Square Breathing

Four count inhale
Four count hold
Four count exhale
Four count hold

Journal one paragraph reflecting upon your day. This is a constructive review. Keep the reflection nonjudgmental.

Example: *Shortcomings and Successes*

I was resentful, selfish, fearful, dishonest.
I was kind, loving, compassionate.
I achieved all my short-term goals but one.

Include: *Where could I have done better? Constructive improvements...*

_____

_____

_____

_____

_____

_____

_____

_____

DAY 44

DATE: _____

1. Five minutes of Square Breathing

   Four count inhale
   Four count hold
   Four count exhale
   Four count hold

2. Emotional intelligence

   Identify the feeling in your body
   Release emotions not serving you

3. Set up to three *being* intentions

   Example: Spiritual or cognitive intention

   I will live in compassion.
   I will live in tolerance.
   I will speak with love.

   My *being* intentions for today are:

   _____
   _____
   _____

4. Set up to three *doing* intentions

   Example: Three short-term goals for the day

   Today, I will clean the house.
   I will run daily errands.
   I will meditate for ten minutes.

   My *doing* intentions for today are:

   _____
   _____
   _____

   Acknowledge your ninety-day goal:

   _____
   _____

5. Fitness/Movement goal

   Example: *one-hour workout, bike ride, thirty-minute dog walk, swim...*

   My fitness/movement goal for today is:

   _____

   Personal Relationships

   Example: *One action to nurture a personal relationship*

   Lunch with friend/coworker
   Movie with partner
   Park with children

   My plan for today to nurture a personal relationship:

   _____

6. Short reflection for the day

_____

_____

_____

_____

_____

7. Five minutes of Square Breathing

   Four count inhale
   Four count hold
   Four count exhale
   Four count hold

   Journal one paragraph reflecting upon your day. This is a constructive review. Keep the reflection nonjudgmental.

   Example: *Shortcomings and Successes*

   I was resentful, selfish, fearful, dishonest.
   I was kind, loving, compassionate.
   I achieved all my short-term goals but one.

   Include: *Where could I have done better? Constructive improvements...*

_____

_____

_____

_____

_____

_____

_____

DAY 45

DATE: _____

1. Five minutes of Square Breathing

   Four count inhale
   Four count hold
   Four count exhale
   Four count hold

2. Emotional intelligence

   Identify the feeling in your body
   Release emotions not serving you

3. Set up to three *being* intentions

   Example: Spiritual or cognitive intention

   I will live in compassion.
   I will live in tolerance.
   I will speak with love.

   My *being* intentions for today are:

   _____

   _____

   _____

4. Set up to three *doing* intentions

   Example: Three short-term goals for the day

   Today, I will clean the house.
   I will run daily errands.
   I will meditate for ten minutes.

   My *doing* intentions for today are:

   _____

   _____

   _____

   Acknowledge your ninety-day goal:

   _____

   _____

5. Fitness/Movement goal

   Example: *one-hour workout, bike ride, thirty-minute dog walk, swim...*

   My fitness/movement goal for today is:

   _____

   Personal Relationships

   Example: *One action to nurture a personal relationship*

   Lunch with friend/coworker
   Movie with partner
   Park with children

   My plan for today to nurture a personal relationship:

   _____

6. Short reflection for the day

_____

_____

_____

_____

_____

7. Five minutes of Square Breathing

Four count inhale
Four count hold
Four count exhale
Four count hold

Journal one paragraph reflecting upon your day.
This is a constructive review. Keep the reflection
nonjudgmental.

Example: *Shortcomings and Successes*

I was resentful, selfish, fearful, dishonest.
I was kind, loving, compassionate.
I achieved all my short-term goals but one.

Include: *Where could I have done better? Constructive*
improvements...

_____

_____

_____

_____

_____

_____

_____

_____

DAY 46

DATE: _____

1. Five minutes of Square Breathing

   Four count inhale
   Four count hold
   Four count exhale
   Four count hold

2. Emotional intelligence

   Identify the feeling in your body
   Release emotions not serving you

3. Set up to three *being* intentions

   Example: Spiritual or cognitive intention

   I will live in compassion.
   I will live in tolerance.
   I will speak with love.

   My *being* intentions for today are:

   _____
   _____
   _____

4. Set up to three *doing* intentions

   Example: Three short-term goals for the day

   Today, I will clean the house.
   I will run daily errands.
   I will meditate for ten minutes.

   My *doing* intentions for today are:

   _____

   _____

   _____

   Acknowledge your ninety-day goal:

   _____

   _____

5. Fitness/Movement goal

   Example: *one-hour workout, bike ride, thirty-minute dog walk, swim...*

   My fitness/movement goal for today is:

   _____

   Personal Relationships

   Example: *One action to nurture a personal relationship*

   Lunch with friend/coworker
   Movie with partner
   Park with children

   My plan for today to nurture a personal relationship:

   _____

6. Short reflection for the day

_____

_____

_____

_____

_____

7. Five minutes of Square Breathing

   Four count inhale
   Four count hold
   Four count exhale
   Four count hold

   Journal one paragraph reflecting upon your day. This is a constructive review. Keep the reflection nonjudgmental.

   Example: _Shortcomings and Successes_

   I was resentful, selfish, fearful, dishonest.
   I was kind, loving, compassionate.
   I achieved all my short-term goals but one.

   Include: _Where could I have done better? Constructive improvements..._

_____

_____

_____

_____

_____

_____

_____

DAY 47

DATE: _____

1. Five minutes of Square Breathing

   Four count inhale
   Four count hold
   Four count exhale
   Four count hold

2. Emotional intelligence

   Identify the feeling in your body
   Release emotions not serving you

3. Set up to three *being* intentions

   Example: Spiritual or cognitive intention

   I will live in compassion.
   I will live in tolerance.
   I will speak with love.

   My *being* intentions for today are:

   _____
   _____
   _____

4. Set up to three *doing* intentions

   Example: Three short-term goals for the day

   Today, I will clean the house.
   I will run daily errands.
   I will meditate for ten minutes.

   My *doing* intentions for today are:

   _____

   _____

   _____

   Acknowledge your ninety-day goal:

   _____

   _____

5. Fitness/Movement goal

   Example: *one-hour workout, bike ride, thirty-minute dog walk, swim...*

   My fitness/movement goal for today is:

   _____

   Personal Relationships

   Example: *One action to nurture a personal relationship*

   Lunch with friend/coworker
   Movie with partner
   Park with children

   My plan for today to nurture a personal relationship:

   _____

6. Short reflection for the day

_____

_____

_____

_____

_____

7. Five minutes of Square Breathing

    Four count inhale
    Four count hold
    Four count exhale
    Four count hold

    Journal one paragraph reflecting upon your day.
    This is a constructive review. Keep the reflection
    nonjudgmental.

    Example: *Shortcomings and Successes*

    I was resentful, selfish, fearful, dishonest.
    I was kind, loving, compassionate.
    I achieved all my short-term goals but one.

    Include: *Where could I have done better? Constructive*
    improvements...

_____

_____

_____

_____

_____

_____

_____

_____

DAY 48

DATE: _____

1. Five minutes of Square Breathing

    Four count inhale
    Four count hold
    Four count exhale
    Four count hold

2. Emotional intelligence

    Identify the feeling in your body
    Release emotions not serving you

3. Set up to three *being* intentions

    Example: Spiritual or cognitive intention

    I will live in compassion.
    I will live in tolerance.
    I will speak with love.

    My *being* intentions for today are:

    _____

    _____

    _____

DAY 48

4. Set up to three *doing* intentions

   Example: Three short-term goals for the day

   Today, I will clean the house.
   I will run daily errands.
   I will meditate for ten minutes.

   My *doing* intentions for today are:

   _____
   _____
   _____

   Acknowledge your ninety-day goal:

   _____
   _____

5. Fitness/Movement goal

   Example: *one-hour workout, bike ride, thirty-minute dog walk, swim...*

   My fitness/movement goal for today is:

   _____

   Personal Relationships

   Example: *One action to nurture a personal relationship*

   Lunch with friend/coworker
   Movie with partner
   Park with children

   My plan for today to nurture a personal relationship:

   _____

6. Short reflection for the day

_____
_____
_____
_____
_____

7. Five minutes of Square Breathing

    Four count inhale
    Four count hold
    Four count exhale
    Four count hold

    Journal one paragraph reflecting upon your day. This is a constructive review. Keep the reflection nonjudgmental.

    Example: *Shortcomings and Successes*

    I was resentful, selfish, fearful, dishonest.
    I was kind, loving, compassionate.
    I achieved all my short-term goals but one.

    Include: *Where could I have done better? Constructive improvements...*

    _____
    _____
    _____
    _____
    _____
    _____
    _____
    _____

DAY 49

DATE: _____

1. Five minutes of Square Breathing

   Four count inhale
   Four count hold
   Four count exhale
   Four count hold

2. Emotional intelligence

   Identify the feeling in your body
   Release emotions not serving you

3. Set up to three *being* intentions

   Example: Spiritual or cognitive intention

   I will live in compassion.
   I will live in tolerance.
   I will speak with love.

   My *being* intentions for today are:

   _____

   _____

   _____

4. Set up to three *doing* intentions

   Example: Three short-term goals for the day

   Today, I will clean the house.
   I will run daily errands.
   I will meditate for ten minutes.

   My *doing* intentions for today are:

   _____

   _____

   _____

   Acknowledge your ninety-day goal:

   _____

   _____

5. Fitness/Movement goal

   Example: *one-hour workout, bike ride, thirty-minute dog walk, swim...*

   My fitness/movement goal for today is:

   _____

   Personal Relationships

   Example: *One action to nurture a personal relationship*

   Lunch with friend/coworker
   Movie with partner
   Park with children

   My plan for today to nurture a personal relationship:

   _____

6. Short reflection for the day

_____

_____

_____

_____

_____

7. Five minutes of Square Breathing

Four count inhale
Four count hold
Four count exhale
Four count hold

Journal one paragraph reflecting upon your day. This is a constructive review. Keep the reflection nonjudgmental.

Example: *Shortcomings and Successes*

I was resentful, selfish, fearful, dishonest.
I was kind, loving, compassionate.
I achieved all my short-term goals but one.

Include: *Where could I have done better? Constructive improvements...*

_____

_____

_____

_____

_____

_____

_____

DAY50

DATE: _____

1. Five minutes of Square Breathing

   Four count inhale
   Four count hold
   Four count exhale
   Four count hold

2. Emotional intelligence

   Identify the feeling in your body
   Release emotions not serving you

3. Set up to three *being* intentions

   Example: Spiritual or cognitive intention

   I will live in compassion.
   I will live in tolerance.
   I will speak with love.

   My *being* intentions for today are:

   _____

   _____

   _____

4. Set up to three *doing* intentions

   Example: Three short-term goals for the day

   Today, I will clean the house.
   I will run daily errands.
   I will meditate for ten minutes.

   My *doing* intentions for today are:

   _____
   _____
   _____

   Acknowledge your ninety-day goal:

   _____
   _____

5. Fitness/Movement goal

   Example: *one-hour workout, bike ride, thirty-minute dog walk, swim...*

   My fitness/movement goal for today is:

   _____

   Personal Relationships

   Example: *One action to nurture a personal relationship*

   Lunch with friend/coworker
   Movie with partner
   Park with children

   My plan for today to nurture a personal relationship:

   _____

6. Short reflection for the day

_____

_____

_____

_____

_____

7. Five minutes of Square Breathing

Four count inhale
Four count hold
Four count exhale
Four count hold

Journal one paragraph reflecting upon your day. This is a constructive review. Keep the reflection nonjudgmental.

Example: *Shortcomings and Successes*

I was resentful, selfish, fearful, dishonest.
I was kind, loving, compassionate.
I achieved all my short-term goals but one.

Include: *Where could I have done better? Constructive improvements...*

_____

_____

_____

_____

_____

_____

_____

_____

DAY 51

DATE: _____

1. Five minutes of Square Breathing

   Four count inhale
   Four count hold
   Four count exhale
   Four count hold

2. Emotional intelligence

   Identify the feeling in your body
   Release emotions not serving you

3. Set up to three *being* intentions

   Example: Spiritual or cognitive intention

   I will live in compassion,
   I will live in tolerance.
   I will speak with love.

   My *being* intentions for today are:

   _____
   _____
   _____

4. Set up to three *doing* intentions

    Example: Three short-term goals for the day

    Today, I will clean the house.
    I will run daily errands.
    I will meditate for ten minutes.

    My *doing* intentions for today are:

    _____

    _____

    _____

    Acknowledge your ninety-day goal:

    _____

    _____

5. Fitness/Movement goal

    Example: *one-hour workout, bike ride, thirty-minute dog walk, swim...*

    My fitness/movement goal for today is:

    _____

    Personal Relationships

    Example: *One action to nurture a personal relationship*

    Lunch with friend/coworker
    Movie with partner
    Park with children

    My plan for today to nurture a personal relationship:

    _____

6. Short reflection for the day

_____

_____

_____

_____

_____

7. Five minutes of Square Breathing

Four count inhale
Four count hold
Four count exhale
Four count hold

Journal one paragraph reflecting upon your day. This is a constructive review. Keep the reflection nonjudgmental.

Example: *Shortcomings and Successes*

I was resentful, selfish, fearful, dishonest.
I was kind, loving, compassionate.
I achieved all my short-term goals but one.

Include: *Where could I have done better? Constructive improvements...*

_____

_____

_____

_____

_____

_____

_____

DAY 52

DATE: _____

1. Five minutes of Square Breathing

   Four count inhale
   Four count hold
   Four count exhale
   Four count hold

2. Emotional intelligence

   Identify the feeling in your body
   Release emotions not serving you

3. Set up to three *being* intentions

   Example: Spiritual or cognitive intention

   I will live in compassion.
   I will live in tolerance.
   I will speak with love.

   My *being* intentions for today are:

   _____
   _____
   _____

4. Set up to three *doing* intentions

   Example: Three short-term goals for the day

   Today, I will clean the house.
   I will run daily errands.
   I will meditate for ten minutes.

   My *doing* intentions for today are:

   _____

   _____

   _____

   Acknowledge your ninety-day goal:

   _____

   _____

5. Fitness/Movement goal

   Example: *one-hour workout, bike ride, thirty-minute dog walk, swim...*

   My fitness/movement goal for today is:

   _____

   Personal Relationships

   Example: *One action to nurture a personal relationship*

   Lunch with friend/coworker
   Movie with partner
   Park with children

   My plan for today to nurture a personal relationship:

   _____

6. Short reflection for the day

———————————————————————
———————————————————————
———————————————————————
———————————————————————
———————————————————————

7. Five minutes of Square Breathing

Four count inhale
Four count hold
Four count exhale
Four count hold

Journal one paragraph reflecting upon your day. This is a constructive review. Keep the reflection nonjudgmental.

Example: *Shortcomings and Successes*

I was resentful, selfish, fearful, dishonest.
I was kind, loving, compassionate.
I achieved all my short-term goals but one.

Include: *Where could I have done better? Constructive improvements...*

———————————————————————
———————————————————————
———————————————————————
———————————————————————
———————————————————————
———————————————————————
———————————————————————
———————————————————————

DAY 53

DATE: _____

1. Five minutes of Square Breathing

   Four count inhale
   Four count hold
   Four count exhale
   Four count hold

2. Emotional intelligence

   Identify the feeling in your body
   Release emotions not serving you

3. Set up to three *being* intentions

   Example: Spiritual or cognitive intention

   I will live in compassion.
   I will live in tolerance.
   I will speak with love.

   My *being* intentions for today are:

   _____

   _____

   _____

4. Set up to three *doing* intentions

   Example: Three short-term goals for the day

   Today, I will clean the house.
   I will run daily errands.
   I will meditate for ten minutes.

   My *doing* intentions for today are:

   _____
   _____
   _____

   Acknowledge your ninety-day goal:

   _____
   _____

5. Fitness/Movement goal

   Example: *one-hour workout, bike ride, thirty-minute dog walk, swim...*

   My fitness/movement goal for today is:

   _____

   Personal Relationships

   Example: *One action to nurture a personal relationship*

   Lunch with friend/coworker
   Movie with partner
   Park with children

   My plan for today to nurture a personal relationship:

   _____

DAY 53

6. Short reflection for the day

_____
_____
_____
_____
_____

7. Five minutes of Square Breathing

Four count inhale
Four count hold
Four count exhale
Four count hold

Journal one paragraph reflecting upon your day. This is a constructive review. Keep the reflection nonjudgmental.

Example: *Shortcomings and Successes*

I was resentful, selfish, fearful, dishonest.
I was kind, loving, compassionate.
I achieved all my short-term goals but one.

Include: *Where could I have done better? Constructive improvements...*

_____
_____
_____
_____
_____
_____
_____

DAY54

DATE: _____

1. Five minutes of Square Breathing

   Four count inhale
   Four count hold
   Four count exhale
   Four count hold

2. Emotional intelligence

   Identify the feeling in your body
   Release emotions not serving you

3. Set up to three *being* intentions

   Example: Spiritual or cognitive intention

   I will live in compassion.
   I will live in tolerance.
   I will speak with love.

   My *being* intentions for today are:

   _____

   _____

   _____

4. Set up to three *doing* intentions

   Example: Three short-term goals for the day

   Today, I will clean the house.
   I will run daily errands.
   I will meditate for ten minutes.

   My *doing* intentions for today are:

   _____
   _____
   _____

   Acknowledge your ninety-day goal:

   _____
   _____

5. Fitness/Movement goal

   Example: *one-hour workout, bike ride, thirty-minute dog walk, swim...*

   My fitness/movement goal for today is:

   _____

   Personal Relationships

   Example: *One action to nurture a personal relationship*

   Lunch with friend/coworker
   Movie with partner
   Park with children

   My plan for today to nurture a personal relationship:

   _____

6. Short reflection for the day

_____

_____

_____

_____

_____

7. Five minutes of Square Breathing

   Four count inhale
   Four count hold
   Four count exhale
   Four count hold

   Journal one paragraph reflecting upon your day. This is a constructive review. Keep the reflection nonjudgmental.

   Example: *Shortcomings and Successes*

   I was resentful, selfish, fearful, dishonest.
   I was kind, loving, compassionate.
   I achieved all my short-term goals but one.

   Include: *Where could I have done better? Constructive improvements...*

_____

_____

_____

_____

_____

_____

_____

_____

DAY55

DATE: _____

1. Five minutes of Square Breathing

   Four count inhale
   Four count hold
   Four count exhale
   Four count hold

2. Emotional intelligence

   Identify the feeling in your body
   Release emotions not serving you

3. Set up to three *being* intentions

   Example: Spiritual or cognitive intention

   I will live in compassion.
   I will live in tolerance.
   I will speak with love.

   My *being* intentions for today are:

   _____

   _____

   _____

4. Set up to three *doing* intentions

   Example: Three short-term goals for the day

   Today, I will clean the house.
   I will run daily errands.
   I will meditate for ten minutes.

   My *doing* intentions for today are:

   _____

   _____

   _____

   Acknowledge your ninety-day goal:

   _____

   _____

5. Fitness/Movement goal

   Example: *one-hour workout, bike ride, thirty-minute dog walk, swim...*

   My fitness/movement goal for today is:

   _____

   Personal Relationships

   Example: *One action to nurture a personal relationship*

   Lunch with friend/coworker
   Movie with partner
   Park with children

   My plan for today to nurture a personal relationship:

   _____

6. Short reflection for the day

_____
_____
_____
_____
_____

7. Five minutes of Square Breathing

Four count inhale
Four count hold
Four count exhale
Four count hold

Journal one paragraph reflecting upon your day. This is a constructive review. Keep the reflection nonjudgmental.

Example: *Shortcomings and Successes*

I was resentful, selfish, fearful, dishonest.
I was kind, loving, compassionate.
I achieved all my short-term goals but one.

Include: *Where could I have done better? Constructive improvements...*

_____
_____
_____
_____
_____
_____
_____
_____

DAY 56

DATE: _____

1. Five minutes of Square Breathing

   Four count inhale
   Four count hold
   Four count exhale
   Four count hold

2. Emotional intelligence

   Identify the feeling in your body
   Release emotions not serving you

3. Set up to three *being* intentions

   Example: Spiritual or cognitive intention

   I will live in compassion.
   I will live in tolerance.
   I will speak with love.

   My *being* intentions for today are:

   _____
   _____
   _____

4. Set up to three *doing* intentions

    Example: Three short-term goals for the day

    Today, I will clean the house.
    I will run daily errands.
    I will meditate for ten minutes.

    My *doing* intentions for today are:

    _____
    _____
    _____

    Acknowledge your ninety-day goal:

    _____
    _____

5. Fitness/Movement goal

    Example: *one-hour workout, bike ride, thirty-minute dog walk, swim...*

    My fitness/movement goal for today is:

    _____

    Personal Relationships

    Example: *One action to nurture a personal relationship*

    Lunch with friend/coworker
    Movie with partner
    Park with children

    My plan for today to nurture a personal relationship:

    _____

6. Short reflection for the day

   _____
   _____
   _____
   _____
   _____

7. Five minutes of Square Breathing

   Four count inhale
   Four count hold
   Four count exhale
   Four count hold

   Journal one paragraph reflecting upon your day.
   This is a constructive review. Keep the reflection
   nonjudgmental.

   Example: *Shortcomings and Successes*

   I was resentful, selfish, fearful, dishonest.
   I was kind, loving, compassionate.
   I achieved all my short-term goals but one.

   Include: *Where could I have done better? Constructive*
   improvements...

   _____
   _____
   _____
   _____
   _____
   _____
   _____
   _____

DAY57

DATE: _____

1. Five minutes of Square Breathing

   Four count inhale
   Four count hold
   Four count exhale
   Four count hold

2. Emotional intelligence

   Identify the feeling in your body
   Release emotions not serving you

3. Set up to three *being* intentions

   Example: Spiritual or cognitive intention

   I will live in compassion.
   I will live in tolerance.
   I will speak with love.

   My *being* intentions for today are:

   _____
   _____
   _____

4. Set up to three *doing* intentions

   Example: Three short-term goals for the day

   Today, I will clean the house.
   I will run daily errands.
   I will meditate for ten minutes.

   My *doing* intentions for today are:

   _____
   _____
   _____

   Acknowledge your ninety-day goal:

   _____
   _____

5. Fitness/Movement goal

   Example: *one-hour workout, bike ride, thirty-minute dog walk, swim...*

   My fitness/movement goal for today is:

   _____

   Personal Relationships

   Example: *One action to nurture a personal relationship*

   Lunch with friend/coworker
   Movie with partner
   Park with children

   My plan for today to nurture a personal relationship:

   _____

6. Short reflection for the day

_____

_____

_____

_____

_____

7. Five minutes of Square Breathing

Four count inhale
Four count hold
Four count exhale
Four count hold

Journal one paragraph reflecting upon your day.
This is a constructive review. Keep the reflection
nonjudgmental.

Example: *Shortcomings and Successes*

I was resentful, selfish, fearful, dishonest.
I was kind, loving, compassionate.
I achieved all my short-term goals but one.

Include: *Where could I have done better? Constructive*
improvements...

_____

_____

_____

_____

_____

_____

_____

DAY 58

DATE: _____

1. Five minutes of Square Breathing

   Four count inhale
   Four count hold
   Four count exhale
   Four count hold

2. Emotional intelligence

   Identify the feeling in your body
   Release emotions not serving you

3. Set up to three *being* intentions

   Example: Spiritual or cognitive intention

   I will live in compassion.
   I will live in tolerance.
   I will speak with love.

   My *being* intentions for today are:

   _____
   _____
   _____

4. Set up to three *doing* intentions

   Example: Three short-term goals for the day

   Today, I will clean the house.
   I will run daily errands.
   I will meditate for ten minutes.

   My *doing* intentions for today are:

   _____
   _____
   _____

   Acknowledge your ninety-day goal:

   _____
   _____

5. Fitness/Movement goal

   Example: *one-hour workout, bike ride, thirty-minute dog walk, swim...*

   My fitness/movement goal for today is:

   _____

   Personal Relationships

   Example: *One action to nurture a personal relationship*

   Lunch with friend/coworker
   Movie with partner
   Park with children

   My plan for today to nurture a personal relationship:

   _____

6. Short reflection for the day

_____

_____

_____

_____

_____

7. Five minutes of Square Breathing

Four count inhale
Four count hold
Four count exhale
Four count hold

Journal one paragraph reflecting upon your day. This is a constructive review. Keep the reflection nonjudgmental.

Example: *Shortcomings and Successes*

I was resentful, selfish, fearful, dishonest.
I was kind, loving, compassionate.
I achieved all my short-term goals but one.

Include: *Where could I have done better? Constructive improvements...*

_____

_____

_____

_____

_____

_____

_____

_____

DAY 59

DATE: _____

1. Five minutes of Square Breathing

   Four count inhale
   Four count hold
   Four count exhale
   Four count hold

2. Emotional intelligence

   Identify the feeling in your body
   Release emotions not serving you

3. Set up to three *being* intentions

   Example: Spiritual or cognitive intention

   I will live in compassion.
   I will live in tolerance.
   I will speak with love.

   My *being* intentions for today are:

   _____
   _____
   _____

4. Set up to three *doing* intentions

   Example: Three short-term goals for the day

   Today, I will clean the house.
   I will run daily errands.
   I will meditate for ten minutes.

   My *doing* intentions for today are:

   _____

   _____

   _____

   Acknowledge your ninety-day goal:

   _____

   _____

5. Fitness/Movement goal

   Example: *one-hour workout, bike ride, thirty-minute dog walk, swim...*

   My fitness/movement goal for today is:

   _____

   Personal Relationships

   Example: *One action to nurture a personal relationship*

   Lunch with friend/coworker
   Movie with partner
   Park with children

   My plan for today to nurture a personal relationship:

   _____

6. Short reflection for the day

_____

_____

_____

_____

_____

7. Five minutes of Square Breathing

Four count inhale
Four count hold
Four count exhale
Four count hold

Journal one paragraph reflecting upon your day. This is a constructive review. Keep the reflection nonjudgmental.

Example: *Shortcomings and Successes*

I was resentful, selfish, fearful, dishonest.
I was kind, loving, compassionate.
I achieved all my short-term goals but one.

Include: *Where could I have done better? Constructive improvements...*

_____

_____

_____

_____

_____

_____

_____

_____

DAY 60

DATE: _____

1. Five minutes of Square Breathing

   Four count inhale
   Four count hold
   Four count exhale
   Four count hold

2. Emotional intelligence

   Identify the feeling in your body
   Release emotions not serving you

3. Set up to three *being* intentions

   Example: Spiritual or cognitive intention

   I will live in compassion.
   I will live in tolerance.
   I will speak with love.

   My *being* intentions for today are:

   _____

   _____

   _____

4. Set up to three *doing* intentions

   Example: Three short-term goals for the day

   Today, I will clean the house.
   I will run daily errands.
   I will meditate for ten minutes.

   My *doing* intentions for today are:

   _____

   _____

   _____

   Acknowledge your ninety-day goal:

   _____

   _____

5. Fitness/Movement goal

   Example: *one-hour workout, bike ride, thirty-minute dog walk, swim...*

   My fitness/movement goal for today is:

   _____

   Personal Relationships

   Example: *One action to nurture a personal relationship*

   Lunch with friend/coworker
   Movie with partner
   Park with children

   My plan for today to nurture a personal relationship:

   _____

6. Short reflection for the day

_____

_____

_____

_____

_____

7. Five minutes of Square Breathing

Four count inhale
Four count hold
Four count exhale
Four count hold

Journal one paragraph reflecting upon your day. This is a constructive review. Keep the reflection nonjudgmental.

Example: *Shortcomings and Successes*

I was resentful, selfish, fearful, dishonest.
I was kind, loving, compassionate.
I achieved all my short-term goals but one.

Include: *Where could I have done better? Constructive improvements…*

_____

_____

_____

_____

_____

_____

_____

DAY 61

DATE: _____

1. Five minutes of Square Breathing

   Four count inhale
   Four count hold
   Four count exhale
   Four count hold

2. Emotional intelligence

   Identify the feeling in your body
   Release emotions not serving you

3. Set up to three *being* intentions

   Example: Spiritual or cognitive intention

   I will live in compassion.
   I will live in tolerance.
   I will speak with love.

   My *being* intentions for today are:

   _____

   _____

   _____

4. Set up to three *doing* intentions

   Example: Three short-term goals for the day

   Today, I will clean the house.
   I will run daily errands.
   I will meditate for ten minutes.

   My *doing* intentions for today are:

   _____
   _____
   _____

   Acknowledge your ninety-day goal:

   _____
   _____

5. Fitness/Movement goal

   Example: *one-hour workout, bike ride, thirty-minute dog walk, swim...*

   My fitness/movement goal for today is:

   _____

   Personal Relationships

   Example: *One action to nurture a personal relationship*

   Lunch with friend/coworker
   Movie with partner
   Park with children

   My plan for today to nurture a personal relationship:

   _____

6. Short reflection for the day

_____

_____

_____

_____

_____

7. Five minutes of Square Breathing

Four count inhale
Four count hold
Four count exhale
Four count hold

Journal one paragraph reflecting upon your day. This is a constructive review. Keep the reflection nonjudgmental.

Example: *Shortcomings and Successes*

I was resentful, selfish, fearful, dishonest.
I was kind, loving, compassionate.
I achieved all my short-term goals but one.

Include: *Where could I have done better? Constructive improvements...*

_____

_____

_____

_____

_____

_____

_____

_____

DAY **62**

DATE: _____

1. Five minutes of Square Breathing

   Four count inhale
   Four count hold
   Four count exhale
   Four count hold

2. Emotional intelligence

   Identify the feeling in your body
   Release emotions not serving you

3. Set up to three *being* intentions

   Example: Spiritual or cognitive intention

   I will live in compassion.
   I will live in tolerance.
   I will speak with love.

   My *being* intentions for today are:

   _____
   _____
   _____

4. Set up to three *doing* intentions

   Example: Three short-term goals for the day

   Today, I will clean the house.
   I will run daily errands.
   I will meditate for ten minutes.

   My *doing* intentions for today are:

   _____

   _____

   _____

   Acknowledge your ninety-day goal:

   _____

   _____

5. Fitness/Movement goal

   Example: *one-hour workout, bike ride, thirty-minute dog walk, swim...*

   My fitness/movement goal for today is:

   _____

   Personal Relationships

   Example: *One action to nurture a personal relationship*

   Lunch with friend/coworker
   Movie with partner
   Park with children

   My plan for today to nurture a personal relationship:

   _____

6. Short reflection for the day

_____
_____
_____
_____
_____

7. Five minutes of Square Breathing

Four count inhale
Four count hold
Four count exhale
Four count hold

Journal one paragraph reflecting upon your day.
This is a constructive review. Keep the reflection
nonjudgmental.

Example: *Shortcomings and Successes*

I was resentful, selfish, fearful, dishonest.
I was kind, loving, compassionate.
I achieved all my short-term goals but one.

Include: *Where could I have done better? Constructive
improvements...*

_____
_____
_____
_____
_____
_____
_____
_____

DAY 63

DATE: _____

1. Five minutes of Square Breathing

   Four count inhale
   Four count hold
   Four count exhale
   Four count hold

2. Emotional intelligence

   Identify the feeling in your body
   Release emotions not serving you

3. Set up to three *being* intentions

   Example: Spiritual or cognitive intention

   I will live in compassion.
   I will live in tolerance.
   I will speak with love.

   My *being* intentions for today are:

   _____

   _____

   _____

4. Set up to three *doing* intentions

   Example: Three short-term goals for the day

   Today, I will clean the house.
   I will run daily errands.
   I will meditate for ten minutes.

   My *doing* intentions for today are:

   _____

   _____

   _____

   Acknowledge your ninety-day goal:

   _____

   _____

5. Fitness/Movement goal

   Example: *one-hour workout, bike ride, thirty-minute dog walk, swim...*

   My fitness/movement goal for today is:

   _____

   Personal Relationships

   Example: *One action to nurture a personal relationship*

   Lunch with friend/coworker
   Movie with partner
   Park with children

   My plan for today to nurture a personal relationship:

   _____

6. Short reflection for the day

_____

_____

_____

_____

_____

7. Five minutes of Square Breathing

Four count inhale
Four count hold
Four count exhale
Four count hold

Journal one paragraph reflecting upon your day. This is a constructive review. Keep the reflection nonjudgmental.

Example: *Shortcomings and Successes*

I was resentful, selfish, fearful, dishonest.
I was kind, loving, compassionate.
I achieved all my short-term goals but one.

Include: *Where could I have done better? Constructive improvements...*

_____

_____

_____

_____

_____

_____

_____

DAY 64

DATE: _____

1. Five minutes of Square Breathing

   Four count inhale
   Four count hold
   Four count exhale
   Four count hold

2. Emotional intelligence

   Identify the feeling in your body
   Release emotions not serving you

3. Set up to three *being* intentions

   Example: Spiritual or cognitive intention

   I will live in compassion.
   I will live in tolerance.
   I will speak with love.

   My *being* intentions for today are:

   _____

   _____

   _____

4. Set up to three *doing* intentions

   Example: Three short-term goals for the day

   Today, I will clean the house.
   I will run daily errands.
   I will meditate for ten minutes.

   My *doing* intentions for today are:

   _____

   _____

   _____

   Acknowledge your ninety-day goal:

   _____

   _____

5. Fitness/Movement goal

   Example: *one-hour workout, bike ride, thirty-minute dog walk, swim...*

   My fitness/movement goal for today is:

   _____

   Personal Relationships

   Example: *One action to nurture a personal relationship*

   Lunch with friend/coworker
   Movie with partner
   Park with children

   My plan for today to nurture a personal relationship:

   _____

6. Short reflection for the day

_____

_____

_____

_____

_____

7. Five minutes of Square Breathing

Four count inhale
Four count hold
Four count exhale
Four count hold

Journal one paragraph reflecting upon your day. This is a constructive review. Keep the reflection nonjudgmental.

Example: *Shortcomings and Successes*

I was resentful, selfish, fearful, dishonest.
I was kind, loving, compassionate.
I achieved all my short-term goals but one.

Include: *Where could I have done better? Constructive improvements...*

_____

_____

_____

_____

_____

_____

_____

_____

DAY65

DATE: _____

1. Five minutes of Square Breathing

   Four count inhale
   Four count hold
   Four count exhale
   Four count hold

2. Emotional intelligence

   Identify the feeling in your body
   Release emotions not serving you

3. Set up to three *being* intentions

   Example: Spiritual or cognitive intention

   I will live in compassion.
   I will live in tolerance.
   I will speak with love.

   My *being* intentions for today are:

   _____
   _____
   _____

4. Set up to three *doing* intentions

   Example: Three short-term goals for the day

   Today, I will clean the house.
   I will run daily errands.
   I will meditate for ten minutes.

   My *doing* intentions for today are:

   _____

   _____

   _____

   Acknowledge your ninety-day goal:

   _____

   _____

5. Fitness/Movement goal

   Example: *one-hour workout, bike ride, thirty-minute dog walk, swim...*

   My fitness/movement goal for today is:

   _____

   Personal Relationships

   Example: *One action to nurture a personal relationship*

   Lunch with friend/coworker
   Movie with partner
   Park with children

   My plan for today to nurture a personal relationship:

   _____

6. Short reflection for the day

_____

_____

_____

_____

_____

7. Five minutes of Square Breathing

Four count inhale
Four count hold
Four count exhale
Four count hold

Journal one paragraph reflecting upon your day. This is a constructive review. Keep the reflection nonjudgmental.

Example: *Shortcomings and Successes*

I was resentful, selfish, fearful, dishonest.
I was kind, loving, compassionate.
I achieved all my short-term goals but one.

Include: *Where could I have done better? Constructive improvements...*

_____

_____

_____

_____

_____

_____

_____

DAY 66

DATE: _____

1. Five minutes of Square Breathing

   Four count inhale
   Four count hold
   Four count exhale
   Four count hold

2. Emotional intelligence

   Identify the feeling in your body
   Release emotions not serving you

3. Set up to three *being* intentions

   Example: Spiritual or cognitive intention

   I will live in compassion.
   I will live in tolerance.
   I will speak with love.

   My *being* intentions for today are:

   _____
   _____
   _____

4. Set up to three *doing* intentions

    Example: Three short-term goals for the day

    Today, I will clean the house.
    I will run daily errands.
    I will meditate for ten minutes.

    My *doing* intentions for today are:

    _____
    _____
    _____

    Acknowledge your ninety-day goal:

    _____
    _____

5. Fitness/Movement goal

    Example: *one-hour workout, bike ride, thirty-minute dog walk, swim...*

    My fitness/movement goal for today is:

    _____

    Personal Relationships

    Example: *One action to nurture a personal relationship*

    Lunch with friend/coworker
    Movie with partner
    Park with children

    My plan for today to nurture a personal relationship:

    _____

6. Short reflection for the day

_____

_____

_____

_____

_____

7. Five minutes of Square Breathing

Four count inhale
Four count hold
Four count exhale
Four count hold

Journal one paragraph reflecting upon your day. This is a constructive review. Keep the reflection nonjudgmental.

Example: *Shortcomings and Successes*

I was resentful, selfish, fearful, dishonest.
I was kind, loving, compassionate.
I achieved all my short-term goals but one.

Include: *Where could I have done better? Constructive improvements...*

_____

_____

_____

_____

_____

_____

_____

DAY 67

DATE: _____

1. Five minutes of Square Breathing

   Four count inhale
   Four count hold
   Four count exhale
   Four count hold

2. Emotional intelligence

   Identify the feeling in your body
   Release emotions not serving you

3. Set up to three *being* intentions

   Example: Spiritual or cognitive intention

   I will live in compassion.
   I will live in tolerance.
   I will speak with love.

   My *being* intentions for today are:

   _____

   _____

   _____

4. Set up to three *doing* intentions

   Example: Three short-term goals for the day

   Today, I will clean the house.
   I will run daily errands.
   I will meditate for ten minutes.

   My *doing* intentions for today are:

   _____

   _____

   _____

   Acknowledge your ninety-day goal:

   _____

   _____

5. Fitness/Movement goal

   Example: *one-hour workout, bike ride, thirty-minute dog walk, swim...*

   My fitness/movement goal for today is:

   _____

   Personal Relationships

   Example: *One action to nurture a personal relationship*

   Lunch with friend/coworker
   Movie with partner
   Park with children

   My plan for today to nurture a personal relationship:

   _____

6. Short reflection for the day

_____
_____
_____
_____
_____

7. Five minutes of Square Breathing

Four count inhale
Four count hold
Four count exhale
Four count hold

Journal one paragraph reflecting upon your day. This is a constructive review. Keep the reflection nonjudgmental.

Example: *Shortcomings and Successes*

I was resentful, selfish, fearful, dishonest.
I was kind, loving, compassionate.
I achieved all my short-term goals but one.

Include: *Where could I have done better? Constructive improvements...*

_____
_____
_____
_____
_____
_____
_____

THINKFIT

DAY 68

DATE: _____

1. Five minutes of Square Breathing

   Four count inhale
   Four count hold
   Four count exhale
   Four count hold

2. Emotional intelligence

   Identify the feeling in your body
   Release emotions not serving you

3. Set up to three *being* intentions

   Example: Spiritual or cognitive intention

   I will live in compassion.
   I will live in tolerance.
   I will speak with love.

   My *being* intentions for today are:

   _____
   _____
   _____

4. Set up to three *doing* intentions

   Example: Three short-term goals for the day

   Today, I will clean the house.
   I will run daily errands.
   I will meditate for ten minutes.

   My *doing* intentions for today are:

   _____

   _____

   _____

   Acknowledge your ninety-day goal:

   _____

   _____

5. Fitness/Movement goal

   Example: *one-hour workout, bike ride, thirty-minute dog walk, swim...*

   My fitness/movement goal for today is:

   _____

   Personal Relationships

   Example: *One action to nurture a personal relationship*

   Lunch with friend/coworker
   Movie with partner
   Park with children

   My plan for today to nurture a personal relationship:

   _____

6. Short reflection for the day

    _____
    _____
    _____
    _____
    _____

7. Five minutes of Square Breathing

    Four count inhale
    Four count hold
    Four count exhale
    Four count hold

    Journal one paragraph reflecting upon your day.
    This is a constructive review. Keep the reflection
    nonjudgmental.

    Example: *Shortcomings and Successes*

    I was resentful, selfish, fearful, dishonest.
    I was kind, loving, compassionate.
    I achieved all my short-term goals but one.

    Include: *Where could I have done better? Constructive*
    improvements...

    _____
    _____
    _____
    _____
    _____
    _____
    _____
    _____

DAY 69

DATE: _____

1. Five minutes of Square Breathing

   Four count inhale
   Four count hold
   Four count exhale
   Four count hold

2. Emotional intelligence

   Identify the feeling in your body
   Release emotions not serving you

3. Set up to three *being* intentions

   Example: Spiritual or cognitive intention

   I will live in compassion.
   I will live in tolerance.
   I will speak with love.

   My *being* intentions for today are:

   _____
   _____
   _____

4. Set up to three *doing* intentions

   Example: Three short-term goals for the day

   Today, I will clean the house.
   I will run daily errands.
   I will meditate for ten minutes.

   My *doing* intentions for today are:

   _____

   _____

   _____

   Acknowledge your ninety-day goal:

   _____

   _____

5. Fitness/Movement goal

   Example: *one-hour workout, bike ride, thirty-minute dog walk, swim...*

   My fitness/movement goal for today is:

   _____

   Personal Relationships

   Example: *One action to nurture a personal relationship*

   Lunch with friend/coworker
   Movie with partner
   Park with children

   My plan for today to nurture a personal relationship:

   _____

6. Short reflection for the day

    _____

    _____

    _____

    _____

    _____

7. Five minutes of Square Breathing

    Four count inhale
    Four count hold
    Four count exhale
    Four count hold

    Journal one paragraph reflecting upon your day. This is a constructive review. Keep the reflection nonjudgmental.

    Example: *Shortcomings and Successes*

    I was resentful, selfish, fearful, dishonest.
    I was kind, loving, compassionate.
    I achieved all my short-term goals but one.

    Include: *Where could I have done better? Constructive improvements...*

    _____

    _____

    _____

    _____

    _____

    _____

    _____

DAY 70

DATE: _____

1. Five minutes of Square Breathing

   Four count inhale
   Four count hold
   Four count exhale
   Four count hold

2. Emotional intelligence

   Identify the feeling in your body
   Release emotions not serving you

3. Set up to three *being* intentions

   Example: Spiritual or cognitive intention

   I will live in compassion.
   I will live in tolerance.
   I will speak with love.

   My *being* intentions for today are:

   _____

   _____

   _____

4. Set up to three *doing* intentions

   Example: Three short-term goals for the day

   Today, I will clean the house.
   I will run daily errands.
   I will meditate for ten minutes.

   My *doing* intentions for today are:

   _____
   _____
   _____

   Acknowledge your ninety-day goal:

   _____
   _____

5. Fitness/Movement goal

   Example: *one-hour workout, bike ride, thirty-minute dog walk, swim...*

   My fitness/movement goal for today is:

   _____

   Personal Relationships

   Example: *One action to nurture a personal relationship*

   Lunch with friend/coworker
   Movie with partner
   Park with children

   My plan for today to nurture a personal relationship:

   _____

6. Short reflection for the day

_____

_____

_____

_____

_____

7. Five minutes of Square Breathing

   Four count inhale
   Four count hold
   Four count exhale
   Four count hold

   Journal one paragraph reflecting upon your day. This is a constructive review. Keep the reflection nonjudgmental.

   Example: *Shortcomings and Successes*

   I was resentful, selfish, fearful, dishonest.
   I was kind, loving, compassionate.
   I achieved all my short-term goals but one.

   Include: *Where could I have done better? Constructive improvements...*

_____

_____

_____

_____

_____

_____

_____

_____

DAY71

DATE: _____

1. Five minutes of Square Breathing

   Four count inhale
   Four count hold
   Four count exhale
   Four count hold

2. Emotional intelligence

   Identify the feeling in your body
   Release emotions not serving you

3. Set up to three *being* intentions

   Example: Spiritual or cognitive intention

   I will live in compassion.
   I will live in tolerance.
   I will speak with love.

   My *being* intentions for today are:

   _____
   _____
   _____

4. Set up to three *doing* intentions

   Example: Three short-term goals for the day

   Today, I will clean the house.
   I will run daily errands.
   I will meditate for ten minutes.

   My *doing* intentions for today are:

   _____

   _____

   _____

   Acknowledge your ninety-day goal:

   _____

   _____

5. Fitness/Movement goal

   Example: *one-hour workout, bike ride, thirty-minute dog walk, swim...*

   My fitness/movement goal for today is:

   _____

   Personal Relationships

   Example: *One action to nurture a personal relationship*

   Lunch with friend/coworker
   Movie with partner
   Park with children

   My plan for today to nurture a personal relationship:

   _____

6. Short reflection for the day

_____
_____
_____
_____
_____

7. Five minutes of Square Breathing

Four count inhale
Four count hold
Four count exhale
Four count hold

Journal one paragraph reflecting upon your day.
This is a constructive review. Keep the reflection
nonjudgmental.

Example: *Shortcomings and Successes*

I was resentful, selfish, fearful, dishonest.
I was kind, loving, compassionate.
I achieved all my short-term goals but one.

Include: *Where could I have done better? Constructive*
improvements...

_____
_____
_____
_____
_____
_____
_____
_____

DAY72

DATE: _____

1. Five minutes of Square Breathing

   Four count inhale
   Four count hold
   Four count exhale
   Four count hold

2. Emotional intelligence

   Identify the feeling in your body
   Release emotions not serving you

3. Set up to three *being* intentions

   Example: Spiritual or cognitive intention

   I will live in compassion.
   I will live in tolerance.
   I will speak with love.

   My *being* intentions for today are:

   _____
   _____
   _____

4. Set up to three *doing* intentions

    Example: Three short-term goals for the day

    Today, I will clean the house.
    I will run daily errands.
    I will meditate for ten minutes.

    My *doing* intentions for today are:

    _____
    _____
    _____

    Acknowledge your ninety-day goal:

    _____
    _____

5. Fitness/Movement goal

    Example: *one-hour workout, bike ride, thirty-minute dog walk, swim...*

    My fitness/movement goal for today is:

    _____

    Personal Relationships

    Example: *One action to nurture a personal relationship*

    Lunch with friend/coworker
    Movie with partner
    Park with children

    My plan for today to nurture a personal relationship:

    _____

6. Short reflection for the day

_____

_____

_____

_____

_____

7. Five minutes of Square Breathing

Four count inhale
Four count hold
Four count exhale
Four count hold

Journal one paragraph reflecting upon your day. This is a constructive review. Keep the reflection nonjudgmental.

Example: *Shortcomings and Successes*

I was resentful, selfish, fearful, dishonest.
I was kind, loving, compassionate.
I achieved all my short-term goals but one.

Include: *Where could I have done better? Constructive improvements...*

_____

_____

_____

_____

_____

_____

_____

_____

DAY**73**

DATE: _____

1. Five minutes of Square Breathing

   Four count inhale
   Four count hold
   Four count exhale
   Four count hold

2. Emotional intelligence

   Identify the feeling in your body
   Release emotions not serving you

3. Set up to three *being* intentions

   Example: Spiritual or cognitive intention

   I will live in compassion.
   I will live in tolerance.
   I will speak with love.

   My *being* intentions for today are:

   _____
   _____
   _____

4. Set up to three *doing* intentions

   Example: Three short-term goals for the day

   Today, I will clean the house.
   I will run daily errands.
   I will meditate for ten minutes.

   My *doing* intentions for today are:

   _____

   _____

   _____

   Acknowledge your ninety-day goal:

   _____

   _____

5. Fitness/Movement goal

   Example: *one-hour workout, bike ride, thirty-minute dog walk, swim...*

   My fitness/movement goal for today is:

   _____

   Personal Relationships

   Example: *One action to nurture a personal relationship*

   Lunch with friend/coworker
   Movie with partner
   Park with children

   My plan for today to nurture a personal relationship:

   _____

6. Short reflection for the day

   _____

   _____

   _____

   _____

   _____

7. Five minutes of Square Breathing

   Four count inhale
   Four count hold
   Four count exhale
   Four count hold

   Journal one paragraph reflecting upon your day.
   This is a constructive review. Keep the reflection
   nonjudgmental.

   Example: *Shortcomings and Successes*

   I was resentful, selfish, fearful, dishonest.
   I was kind, loving, compassionate.
   I achieved all my short-term goals but one.

   Include: *Where could I have done better? Constructive*
   improvements...

   _____

   _____

   _____

   _____

   _____

   _____

   _____

   _____

DAY74

DATE: _____

1. Five minutes of Square Breathing

   Four count inhale
   Four count hold
   Four count exhale
   Four count hold

2. Emotional intelligence

   Identify the feeling in your body
   Release emotions not serving you

3. Set up to three *being* intentions

   Example: Spiritual or cognitive intention

   I will live in compassion.
   I will live in tolerance.
   I will speak with love.

   My *being* intentions for today are:

   _____
   _____
   _____

DAY 74

4. Set up to three *doing* intentions

   Example: Three short-term goals for the day

   Today, I will clean the house.
   I will run daily errands.
   I will meditate for ten minutes.

   My *doing* intentions for today are:

   _____
   _____
   _____

   Acknowledge your ninety-day goal:

   _____
   _____

5. Fitness/Movement goal

   Example: *one-hour workout, bike ride, thirty-minute dog walk, swim...*

   My fitness/movement goal for today is:

   _____

   Personal Relationships

   Example: *One action to nurture a personal relationship*

   Lunch with friend/coworker
   Movie with partner
   Park with children

   My plan for today to nurture a personal relationship:

   _____

6. Short reflection for the day

   _____

   _____

   _____

   _____

   _____

7. Five minutes of Square Breathing

   Four count inhale
   Four count hold
   Four count exhale
   Four count hold

   Journal one paragraph reflecting upon your day. This is a constructive review. Keep the reflection nonjudgmental.

   Example: *Shortcomings and Successes*

   I was resentful, selfish, fearful, dishonest.
   I was kind, loving, compassionate.
   I achieved all my short-term goals but one.

   Include: *Where could I have done better? Constructive improvements...*

   _____

   _____

   _____

   _____

   _____

   _____

   _____

   _____

DAY75

DATE: _____

1. Five minutes of Square Breathing

   Four count inhale
   Four count hold
   Four count exhale
   Four count hold

2. Emotional intelligence

   Identify the feeling in your body
   Release emotions not serving you

3. Set up to three *being* intentions

   Example: Spiritual or cognitive intention

   I will live in compassion.
   I will live in tolerance.
   I will speak with love.

   My *being* intentions for today are:

   _____
   _____
   _____

4. Set up to three *doing* intentions

   Example: Three short-term goals for the day

   Today, I will clean the house.
   I will run daily errands.
   I will meditate for ten minutes.

   My *doing* intentions for today are:

   _____

   _____

   _____

   Acknowledge your ninety-day goal:

   _____

   _____

5. Fitness/Movement goal

   Example: *one-hour workout, bike ride, thirty-minute dog walk, swim...*

   My fitness/movement goal for today is:

   _____

   Personal Relationships

   Example: *One action to nurture a personal relationship*

   Lunch with friend/coworker
   Movie with partner
   Park with children

   My plan for today to nurture a personal relationship:

   _____

6. Short reflection for the day

_____

_____

_____

_____

_____

7. Five minutes of Square Breathing

   Four count inhale
   Four count hold
   Four count exhale
   Four count hold

   Journal one paragraph reflecting upon your day.
   This is a constructive review. Keep the reflection
   nonjudgmental.

   Example: *Shortcomings and Successes*

   I was resentful, selfish, fearful, dishonest.
   I was kind, loving, compassionate.
   I achieved all my short-term goals but one.

   Include: *Where could I have done better? Constructive*
   improvements...

   _____

   _____

   _____

   _____

   _____

   _____

   _____

DAY76

DATE: _____

1. Five minutes of Square Breathing

   Four count inhale
   Four count hold
   Four count exhale
   Four count hold

2. Emotional intelligence

   Identify the feeling in your body
   Release emotions not serving you

3. Set up to three *being* intentions

   Example: Spiritual or cognitive intention

   I will live in compassion.
   I will live in tolerance.
   I will speak with love.

   My *being* intentions for today are:

   _____
   _____
   _____

4. Set up to three *doing* intentions

Example: Three short-term goals for the day

Today, I will clean the house.
I will run daily errands.
I will meditate for ten minutes.

My *doing* intentions for today are:

_____

_____

_____

Acknowledge your ninety-day goal:

_____

_____

5. Fitness/Movement goal

Example: *one-hour workout, bike ride, thirty-minute dog walk, swim...*

My fitness/movement goal for today is:

_____

Personal Relationships

Example: *One action to nurture a personal relationship*

Lunch with friend/coworker
Movie with partner
Park with children

My plan for today to nurture a personal relationship:

_____

6. Short reflection for the day

_____

_____

_____

_____

_____

7. Five minutes of Square Breathing

Four count inhale
Four count hold
Four count exhale
Four count hold

Journal one paragraph reflecting upon your day. This is a constructive review. Keep the reflection nonjudgmental.

Example: *Shortcomings and Successes*

I was resentful, selfish, fearful, dishonest.
I was kind, loving, compassionate.
I achieved all my short-term goals but one.

Include: *Where could I have done better? Constructive improvements...*

_____

_____

_____

_____

_____

_____

_____

_____

DAY77

DATE: _____

1. Five minutes of Square Breathing

   Four count inhale
   Four count hold
   Four count exhale
   Four count hold

2. Emotional intelligence

   Identify the feeling in your body
   Release emotions not serving you

3. Set up to three *being* intentions

   Example: Spiritual or cognitive intention

   I will live in compassion.
   I will live in tolerance.
   I will speak with love.

   My *being* intentions for today are:

   _____

   _____

   _____

4. Set up to three *doing* intentions

    Example: Three short-term goals for the day

    Today, I will clean the house.
    I will run daily errands.
    I will meditate for ten minutes.

    My *doing* intentions for today are:

    _____
    _____
    _____

    Acknowledge your ninety-day goal:

    _____
    _____

5. Fitness/Movement goal

    Example: *one-hour workout, bike ride, thirty-minute dog walk, swim...*

    My fitness/movement goal for today is:

    _____

    Personal Relationships

    Example: *One action to nurture a personal relationship*

    Lunch with friend/coworker
    Movie with partner
    Park with children

    My plan for today to nurture a personal relationship:

    _____

DAY 77

6. Short reflection for the day

    _____

    _____

    _____

    _____

    _____

7. Five minutes of Square Breathing

    Four count inhale
    Four count hold
    Four count exhale
    Four count hold

    Journal one paragraph reflecting upon your day.
    This is a constructive review. Keep the reflection
    nonjudgmental.

    Example: *Shortcomings and Successes*

    I was resentful, selfish, fearful, dishonest.
    I was kind, loving, compassionate.
    I achieved all my short-term goals but one.

    Include: *Where could I have done better? Constructive*
    improvements...

    _____

    _____

    _____

    _____

    _____

    _____

    _____

    _____

DAY78

DATE: _____

1. Five minutes of Square Breathing

   Four count inhale
   Four count hold
   Four count exhale
   Four count hold

2. Emotional intelligence

   Identify the feeling in your body
   Release emotions not serving you

3. Set up to three *being* intentions

   Example: Spiritual or cognitive intention

   I will live in compassion.
   I will live in tolerance.
   I will speak with love.

   My *being* intentions for today are:

   _____

   _____

   _____

4. Set up to three *doing* intentions

   Example: Three short-term goals for the day

   Today, I will clean the house.
   I will run daily errands.
   I will meditate for ten minutes.

   My *doing* intentions for today are:

   _____
   _____
   _____

   Acknowledge your ninety-day goal:

   _____
   _____

5. Fitness/Movement goal

   Example: *one-hour workout, bike ride, thirty-minute dog walk, swim...*

   My fitness/movement goal for today is:

   _____

   Personal Relationships

   Example: *One action to nurture a personal relationship*

   Lunch with friend/coworker
   Movie with partner
   Park with children

   My plan for today to nurture a personal relationship:

   _____

6. Short reflection for the day

_____

_____

_____

_____

_____

7. Five minutes of Square Breathing

Four count inhale
Four count hold
Four count exhale
Four count hold

Journal one paragraph reflecting upon your day. This is a constructive review. Keep the reflection nonjudgmental.

Example: _Shortcomings and Successes_

I was resentful, selfish, fearful, dishonest.
I was kind, loving, compassionate.
I achieved all my short-term goals but one.

Include: _Where could I have done better? Constructive improvements..._

_____

_____

_____

_____

_____

_____

_____

DAY79

DATE: _____

1. Five minutes of Square Breathing

   Four count inhale
   Four count hold
   Four count exhale
   Four count hold

2. Emotional intelligence

   Identify the feeling in your body
   Release emotions not serving you

3. Set up to three *being* intentions

   Example: Spiritual or cognitive intention

   I will live in compassion.
   I will live in tolerance.
   I will speak with love.

   My *being* intentions for today are:

   _____
   _____
   _____

4. Set up to three *doing* intentions

   Example: Three short-term goals for the day

   Today, I will clean the house.
   I will run daily errands.
   I will meditate for ten minutes.

   My *doing* intentions for today are:

   _____
   _____
   _____

   Acknowledge your ninety-day goal:

   _____
   _____

5. Fitness/Movement goal

   Example: *one-hour workout, bike ride, thirty-minute dog walk, swim...*

   My fitness/movement goal for today is:

   _____

   Personal Relationships

   Example: *One action to nurture a personal relationship*

   Lunch with friend/coworker
   Movie with partner
   Park with children

   My plan for today to nurture a personal relationship:

   _____

6. Short reflection for the day

_____
_____
_____
_____
_____

7. Five minutes of Square Breathing

Four count inhale
Four count hold
Four count exhale
Four count hold

Journal one paragraph reflecting upon your day. This is a constructive review. Keep the reflection nonjudgmental.

Example: *Shortcomings and Successes*

I was resentful, selfish, fearful, dishonest.
I was kind, loving, compassionate.
I achieved all my short-term goals but one.

Include: *Where could I have done better? Constructive improvements...*

_____
_____
_____
_____
_____
_____
_____

DAY 80

DATE: _____

1. Five minutes of Square Breathing

   Four count inhale
   Four count hold
   Four count exhale
   Four count hold

2. Emotional intelligence

   Identify the feeling in your body
   Release emotions not serving you

3. Set up to three *being* intentions

   Example: Spiritual or cognitive intention

   I will live in compassion.
   I will live in tolerance.
   I will speak with love.

   My *being* intentions for today are:

   _____

   _____

   _____

4. Set up to three *doing* intentions

   Example: Three short-term goals for the day

   Today, I will clean the house.
   I will run daily errands.
   I will meditate for ten minutes.

   My *doing* intentions for today are:

   _____
   _____
   _____

   Acknowledge your ninety-day goal:

   _____
   _____

5. Fitness/Movement goal

   Example: *one-hour workout, bike ride, thirty-minute dog walk, swim...*

   My fitness/movement goal for today is:

   _____

   Personal Relationships

   Example: *One action to nurture a personal relationship*

   Lunch with friend/coworker
   Movie with partner
   Park with children

   My plan for today to nurture a personal relationship:

   _____

6. Short reflection for the day

    _____

    _____

    _____

    _____

    _____

7. Five minutes of Square Breathing

    Four count inhale
    Four count hold
    Four count exhale
    Four count hold

    Journal one paragraph reflecting upon your day. This is a constructive review. Keep the reflection nonjudgmental.

    Example: *Shortcomings and Successes*

    I was resentful, selfish, fearful, dishonest.
    I was kind, loving, compassionate.
    I achieved all my short-term goals but one.

    Include: *Where could I have done better? Constructive improvements...*

    _____

    _____

    _____

    _____

    _____

    _____

    _____

DAY 81

DATE: _____

1. Five minutes of Square Breathing

   Four count inhale
   Four count hold
   Four count exhale
   Four count hold

2. Emotional intelligence

   Identify the feeling in your body
   Release emotions not serving you

3. Set up to three *being* intentions

   Example: Spiritual or cognitive intention

   I will live in compassion.
   I will live in tolerance.
   I will speak with love.

   My *being* intentions for today are:

   _____
   _____
   _____

4. Set up to three *doing* intentions

   Example: Three short-term goals for the day

   Today, I will clean the house.
   I will run daily errands.
   I will meditate for ten minutes.

   My *doing* intentions for today are:

   _____

   _____

   _____

   Acknowledge your ninety-day goal:

   _____

   _____

5. Fitness/Movement goal

   Example: *one-hour workout, bike ride, thirty-minute dog walk, swim...*

   My fitness/movement goal for today is:

   _____

   Personal Relationships

   Example: *One action to nurture a personal relationship*

   Lunch with friend/coworker
   Movie with partner
   Park with children

   My plan for today to nurture a personal relationship:

   _____

6. Short reflection for the day

_____
_____
_____
_____
_____

7. Five minutes of Square Breathing

   Four count inhale
   Four count hold
   Four count exhale
   Four count hold

   Journal one paragraph reflecting upon your day. This is a constructive review. Keep the reflection nonjudgmental.

   Example: *Shortcomings and Successes*

   I was resentful, selfish, fearful, dishonest.
   I was kind, loving, compassionate.
   I achieved all my short-term goals but one.

   Include: *Where could I have done better? Constructive improvements...*

_____
_____
_____
_____
_____
_____
_____

DAY82

DATE: _____

1. Five minutes of Square Breathing

   Four count inhale
   Four count hold
   Four count exhale
   Four count hold

2. Emotional intelligence

   Identify the feeling in your body
   Release emotions not serving you

3. Set up to three *being* intentions

   Example: Spiritual or cognitive intention

   I will live in compassion.
   I will live in tolerance.
   I will speak with love.

   My *being* intentions for today are:

   _____
   _____
   _____

4. Set up to three *doing* intentions

   Example: Three short-term goals for the day

   Today, I will clean the house.
   I will run daily errands.
   I will meditate for ten minutes.

   My *doing* intentions for today are:

   _____

   _____

   _____

   Acknowledge your ninety-day goal:

   _____

   _____

5. Fitness/Movement goal

   Example: *one-hour workout, bike ride, thirty-minute dog walk, swim...*

   My fitness/movement goal for today is:

   _____

   Personal Relationships

   Example: *One action to nurture a personal relationship*

   Lunch with friend/coworker
   Movie with partner
   Park with children

   My plan for today to nurture a personal relationship:

   _____

6. Short reflection for the day

_____

_____

_____

_____

_____

7. Five minutes of Square Breathing

Four count inhale
Four count hold
Four count exhale
Four count hold

Journal one paragraph reflecting upon your day. This is a constructive review. Keep the reflection nonjudgmental.

Example: *Shortcomings and Successes*

I was resentful, selfish, fearful, dishonest.
I was kind, loving, compassionate.
I achieved all my short-term goals but one.

Include: *Where could I have done better? Constructive improvements...*

_____

_____

_____

_____

_____

_____

_____

_____

DAY83

DATE: _____

1. Five minutes of Square Breathing

   Four count inhale
   Four count hold
   Four count exhale
   Four count hold

2. Emotional intelligence

   Identify the feeling in your body
   Release emotions not serving you

3. Set up to three *being* intentions

   Example: Spiritual or cognitive intention

   I will live in compassion.
   I will live in tolerance.
   I will speak with love.

   My *being* intentions for today are:

   _____
   _____
   _____

4. Set up to three *doing* intentions

   Example: Three short-term goals for the day

   Today, I will clean the house.
   I will run daily errands.
   I will meditate for ten minutes.

   My *doing* intentions for today are:

   _____

   _____

   _____

   Acknowledge your ninety-day goal:

   _____

   _____

5. Fitness/Movement goal

   Example: *one-hour workout, bike ride, thirty-minute dog walk, swim...*

   My fitness/movement goal for today is:

   _____

   Personal Relationships

   Example: *One action to nurture a personal relationship*

   Lunch with friend/coworker
   Movie with partner
   Park with children

   My plan for today to nurture a personal relationship:

   _____

6. Short reflection for the day

_____

_____

_____

_____

_____

7. Five minutes of Square Breathing

   Four count inhale
   Four count hold
   Four count exhale
   Four count hold

   Journal one paragraph reflecting upon your day. This is a constructive review. Keep the reflection nonjudgmental.

   Example: *Shortcomings and Successes*

   I was resentful, selfish, fearful, dishonest.
   I was kind, loving, compassionate.
   I achieved all my short-term goals but one.

   Include: *Where could I have done better? Constructive improvements...*

_____

_____

_____

_____

_____

_____

_____

_____

DAY84

DATE: _____

1. Five minutes of Square Breathing

   Four count inhale
   Four count hold
   Four count exhale
   Four count hold

2. Emotional intelligence

   Identify the feeling in your body
   Release emotions not serving you

3. Set up to three *being* intentions

   Example: Spiritual or cognitive intention

   I will live in compassion.
   I will live in tolerance.
   I will speak with love.

   My *being* intentions for today are:

   _____
   _____
   _____

4. Set up to three *doing* intentions

    Example: Three short-term goals for the day

    Today, I will clean the house.
    I will run daily errands.
    I will meditate for ten minutes.

    My *doing* intentions for today are:

    _____
    _____
    _____

    Acknowledge your ninety-day goal:

    _____
    _____

5. Fitness/Movement goal

    Example: *one-hour workout, bike ride, thirty-minute dog walk, swim...*

    My fitness/movement goal for today is:

    _____

    Personal Relationships

    Example: *One action to nurture a personal relationship*

    Lunch with friend/coworker
    Movie with partner
    Park with children

    My plan for today to nurture a personal relationship:

    _____

6. Short reflection for the day

_____

_____

_____

_____

_____

7. Five minutes of Square Breathing

   Four count inhale
   Four count hold
   Four count exhale
   Four count hold

   Journal one paragraph reflecting upon your day. This is a constructive review. Keep the reflection nonjudgmental.

   Example: *Shortcomings and Successes*

   I was resentful, selfish, fearful, dishonest.
   I was kind, loving, compassionate.
   I achieved all my short-term goals but one.

   Include: *Where could I have done better? Constructive improvements...*

_____

_____

_____

_____

_____

_____

_____

_____

DAY 85

DATE: _____

1. Five minutes of Square Breathing

   Four count inhale
   Four count hold
   Four count exhale
   Four count hold

2. Emotional intelligence

   Identify the feeling in your body
   Release emotions not serving you

3. Set up to three *being* intentions

   Example: Spiritual or cognitive intention

   I will live in compassion.
   I will live in tolerance.
   I will speak with love.

   My *being* intentions for today are:

   _____

   _____

   _____

4. Set up to three *doing* intentions

   Example: Three short-term goals for the day

   Today, I will clean the house.
   I will run daily errands.
   I will meditate for ten minutes.

   My *doing* intentions for today are:

   _____
   _____
   _____

   Acknowledge your ninety-day goal:

   _____
   _____

5. Fitness/Movement goal

   Example: *one-hour workout, bike ride, thirty-minute dog walk, swim...*

   My fitness/movement goal for today is:

   _____

   Personal Relationships

   Example: *One action to nurture a personal relationship*

   Lunch with friend/coworker
   Movie with partner
   Park with children

   My plan for today to nurture a personal relationship:

   _____

6. Short reflection for the day

_____

_____

_____

_____

_____

7. Five minutes of Square Breathing

Four count inhale
Four count hold
Four count exhale
Four count hold

Journal one paragraph reflecting upon your day. This is a constructive review. Keep the reflection nonjudgmental.

Example: *Shortcomings and Successes*

I was resentful, selfish, fearful, dishonest.
I was kind, loving, compassionate.
I achieved all my short-term goals but one.

Include: *Where could I have done better? Constructive improvements...*

_____

_____

_____

_____

_____

_____

_____

DAY86

DATE: _____

1. Five minutes of Square Breathing

   Four count inhale
   Four count hold
   Four count exhale
   Four count hold

2. Emotional intelligence

   Identify the feeling in your body
   Release emotions not serving you

3. Set up to three *being* intentions

   Example: Spiritual or cognitive intention

   I will live in compassion.
   I will live in tolerance.
   I will speak with love.

   My *being* intentions for today are:

   _____
   _____
   _____

4. Set up to three *doing* intentions

Example: Three short-term goals for the day

Today, I will clean the house.
I will run daily errands.
I will meditate for ten minutes.

My *doing* intentions for today are:

_____
_____
_____

Acknowledge your ninety-day goal:

_____
_____

5. Fitness/Movement goal

Example: *one-hour workout, bike ride, thirty-minute dog walk, swim...*

My fitness/movement goal for today is:

_____

Personal Relationships

Example: *One action to nurture a personal relationship*

Lunch with friend/coworker
Movie with partner
Park with children

My plan for today to nurture a personal relationship:

_____

6. Short reflection for the day

_____
_____
_____
_____
_____

7. Five minutes of Square Breathing

Four count inhale
Four count hold
Four count exhale
Four count hold

Journal one paragraph reflecting upon your day. This is a constructive review. Keep the reflection nonjudgmental.

Example: *Shortcomings and Successes*

I was resentful, selfish, fearful, dishonest.
I was kind, loving, compassionate.
I achieved all my short-term goals but one.

Include: *Where could I have done better? Constructive improvements...*

_____
_____
_____
_____
_____
_____
_____
_____

DAY 87

DATE: _____

1. Five minutes of Square Breathing

   Four count inhale
   Four count hold
   Four count exhale
   Four count hold

2. Emotional intelligence

   Identify the feeling in your body
   Release emotions not serving you

3. Set up to three *being* intentions

   Example: Spiritual or cognitive intention

   I will live in compassion.
   I will live in tolerance.
   I will speak with love.

   My *being* intentions for today are:

   _____
   _____
   _____

4. Set up to three *doing* intentions

   Example: Three short-term goals for the day

   Today, I will clean the house.
   I will run daily errands.
   I will meditate for ten minutes.

   My *doing* intentions for today are:

   _____
   _____
   _____

   Acknowledge your ninety-day goal:

   _____
   _____

5. Fitness/Movement goal

   Example: *one-hour workout, bike ride, thirty-minute dog walk, swim...*

   My fitness/movement goal for today is:

   _____

   Personal Relationships

   Example: *One action to nurture a personal relationship*

   Lunch with friend/coworker
   Movie with partner
   Park with children

   My plan for today to nurture a personal relationship:

   _____

6. Short reflection for the day

_____

_____

_____

_____

_____

7. Five minutes of Square Breathing

Four count inhale
Four count hold
Four count exhale
Four count hold

Journal one paragraph reflecting upon your day. This is a constructive review. Keep the reflection nonjudgmental.

Example: *Shortcomings and Successes*

I was resentful, selfish, fearful, dishonest.
I was kind, loving, compassionate.
I achieved all my short-term goals but one.

Include: *Where could I have done better? Constructive improvements...*

_____

_____

_____

_____

_____

_____

_____

DAY88

DATE: _____

1. Five minutes of Square Breathing

   Four count inhale
   Four count hold
   Four count exhale
   Four count hold

2. Emotional intelligence

   Identify the feeling in your body
   Release emotions not serving you

3. Set up to three *being* intentions

   Example: Spiritual or cognitive intention

   I will live in compassion.
   I will live in tolerance.
   I will speak with love.

   My *being* intentions for today are:

   _____
   _____
   _____

4. Set up to three *doing* intentions

   Example: Three short-term goals for the day

   Today, I will clean the house.
   I will run daily errands.
   I will meditate for ten minutes.

   My *doing* intentions for today are:

   _____

   _____

   _____

   Acknowledge your ninety-day goal:

   _____

   _____

5. Fitness/Movement goal

   Example: *one-hour workout, bike ride, thirty-minute dog walk, swim...*

   My fitness/movement goal for today is:

   _____

   Personal Relationships

   Example: *One action to nurture a personal relationship*

   Lunch with friend/coworker
   Movie with partner
   Park with children

   My plan for today to nurture a personal relationship:

   _____

6. Short reflection for the day

_____

_____

_____

_____

_____

7. Five minutes of Square Breathing

Four count inhale
Four count hold
Four count exhale
Four count hold

Journal one paragraph reflecting upon your day. This is a constructive review. Keep the reflection nonjudgmental.

Example: *Shortcomings and Successes*

I was resentful, selfish, fearful, dishonest.
I was kind, loving, compassionate.
I achieved all my short-term goals but one.

Include: *Where could I have done better? Constructive improvements...*

_____

_____

_____

_____

_____

_____

_____

DAY89

DATE: _____

1. Five minutes of Square Breathing

   Four count inhale
   Four count hold
   Four count exhale
   Four count hold

2. Emotional intelligence

   Identify the feeling in your body
   Release emotions not serving you

3. Set up to three *being* intentions

   Example: Spiritual or cognitive intention

   I will live in compassion.
   I will live in tolerance.
   I will speak with love.

   My *being* intentions for today are:

   _____

   _____

   _____

4. Set up to three *doing* intentions

   Example: Three short-term goals for the day

   Today, I will clean the house.
   I will run daily errands.
   I will meditate for ten minutes.

   My *doing* intentions for today are:

   _____

   _____

   _____

   Acknowledge your ninety-day goal:

   _____

   _____

5. Fitness/Movement goal

   Example: *one-hour workout, bike ride, thirty-minute dog walk, swim...*

   My fitness/movement goal for today is:

   _____

   Personal Relationships

   Example: *One action to nurture a personal relationship*

   Lunch with friend/coworker
   Movie with partner
   Park with children

   My plan for today to nurture a personal relationship:

   _____

6. Short reflection for the day

_____
_____
_____
_____
_____

7. Five minutes of Square Breathing

Four count inhale
Four count hold
Four count exhale
Four count hold

Journal one paragraph reflecting upon your day.
This is a constructive review. Keep the reflection
nonjudgmental.

Example: *Shortcomings and Successes*

I was resentful, selfish, fearful, dishonest.
I was kind, loving, compassionate.
I achieved all my short-term goals but one.

Include: *Where could I have done better? Constructive
improvements...*

_____
_____
_____
_____
_____
_____
_____
_____

DAY 90

DATE: _____

1. Five minutes of Square Breathing

   Four count inhale
   Four count hold
   Four count exhale
   Four count hold

2. Emotional intelligence

   Identify the feeling in your body
   Release emotions not serving you

3. Set up to three *being* intentions

   Example: Spiritual or cognitive intention

   I will live in compassion.
   I will live in tolerance.
   I will speak with love.

   My *being* intentions for today are:

   _____
   _____
   _____

4. Set up to three *doing* intentions

   Example: Three short-term goals for the day

   Today, I will clean the house.
   I will run daily errands.
   I will meditate for ten minutes.

   My *doing* intentions for today are:

   _____

   _____

   _____

   Acknowledge your ninety-day goal:

   _____

   _____

5. Fitness/Movement goal

   Example: *one-hour workout, bike ride, thirty-minute dog walk, swim...*

   My fitness/movement goal for today is:

   _____

   Personal Relationships

   Example: *One action to nurture a personal relationship*

   Lunch with friend/coworker
   Movie with partner
   Park with children

   My plan for today to nurture a personal relationship:

   _____

6. Short reflection for the day

   _____

   _____

   _____

   _____

   _____

7. Five minutes of Square Breathing

   Four count inhale
   Four count hold
   Four count exhale
   Four count hold

   Journal one paragraph reflecting upon your day. This is a constructive review. Keep the reflection nonjudgmental.

   Example: _Shortcomings and Successes_

   I was resentful, selfish, fearful, dishonest.
   I was kind, loving, compassionate.
   I achieved all my short-term goals but one.

   Include: _Where could I have done better? Constructive improvements..._

   _____

   _____

   _____

   _____

   _____

   _____

   _____

   _____

ABOUT THE AUTHOR

Eric Rias, a Queens native, has experienced much of what life has to offer, both good and bad, in just a few short years. As the middle child of accomplished parents, he found himself struggling with self-esteem and issues fitting in. These struggles led him to a cycle of addiction through his early twenties.

After moving to Southern California in 2013, Eric transformed his life. Today, he dedicates himself to transforming the lives of others. In his sobriety, he has helped many individuals achieve their health and wellness goals, while drawing upon his background in personal training, nutrition, and recovery. He wrote *Thinkfit* to guide individuals through his comprehensive coaching programs where he incorporates nutrition and movement while acknowledging emotional and cognitive blocks. The foundation of Eric's programs is based in the understanding that in order to continue to excel, one's main focus must be serving others.

THINKFIT

For a complimentary vision call with Eric,
email eric.thinkfitcoach@gmail.com

For media bookings, email eric.thinkfitcoach@gmail.com

You are also invited to follow Eric's journey at:
Instagram: eric_thinkfitcoach
Facebook: thinkfitsd
Website: thinkfitsd.com

Finally, to stay in tune with health and wellness culture and to get to know more about Eric, follow his podcast *Hearts and Minds Collective* on iTunes, Spotify, and YouTube.

Made in the USA
Middletown, DE
05 September 2019